# When Your Pet Dies

This understanding companion can help you overcome your grief, with inspiring personal insights and words of comfort on . . .

- Why pets are so important
- Roles pets play in the lives of their human companions
- Different ways people grieve
- Stages of grief
- Coping with grief
- When your pet dies suddenly
- When your pet dies after a long illness
- Dealing with the pain of euthanasia
- Caring for your pet's remains
- Helping children, the elderly, and people with disabilities deal with loss
- When other pets suffer over loss
- Involuntary or difficult separations
- How to decide when you are ready to adopt a new pet
- Considerations when choosing a new pet

Appendices include address and telephone lists of helpful national organizations, on-line computer services, support groups, hotlines, pet bereavement counselors, pet cemeteries, plus lists of relevant books and videos for both children and adults.

*Christine Adamec has loved and lost turtles, dogs, and cats. The author of three nonfiction books and more than eight hundred magazine and newspaper articles, she lives in Palm Bay, Florida, with her husband, John, their three children, Jane, Brian and Stephen, and their cats, Miss Kitty and Cleo.*

# When Your Pet Dies

## Christine Adamec

**B**

BERKLEY BOOKS, NEW YORK

## WHEN YOUR PET DIES

A Berkley Book / published by arrangement with
the author

PRINTING HISTORY
Berkley edition / April 1996

ISBN: 0-425-15253-7

BERKLEY®
Berkley Books are published by The Berkley Publishing Group,
200 Madison Avenue, New York, New York 10016.
BERKLEY and the "B" design
are trademarks belonging to Berkley Publishing Corporation.

PRINTED IN THE UNITED STATES OF AMERICA

10  9  8  7  6  5  4  3  2  1

# *Acknowledgments*

I'd like to thank John Adamec, my husband and best friend, for his constant and caring support as I researched and wrote this book. And I certainly think it's important to mention here that John is one of the few people I know who *has* given his secretary time off when her dog died. He is also cocompanion with me to our cats, Miss Kitty and Cleo. Quite a rare human!

I'd also like to thank the many people I interviewed and without whom this book would not have been possible. The professionals provided me with acutely insightful and practical tips and the bereaved pet owners gave me an up-close and personal look at how they perceived their grief as well as their compassionate recommendations for others.

In addition, much thanks goes to the library staff at the DeGroodt Library in Palm Bay, Florida, particularly the following people: Megan McDonald, head of reference, Marie Faure, reference librarian, and Pam Hobson, reference assistant. In addition, Shirley Welch, interlibrary loan librarian at the Central Brevard Library and Reference Center in Cocoa, Florida, provided tremendous assistance in obtaining the books and journal articles I needed. These wonderful ladies worked very hard to fill my endless requests for information, no matter how obscure the source! I appreciate them all very much.

Finally, and very importantly, I would like to thank my editor, Jennifer Lata, for her valuable suggestions.

# *The Rainbow Bridge*

There is a bridge connecting heaven and earth. It is called the Rainbow Bridge, because of its many colors. Just this side of the Rainbow Bridge there is a land of meadows, hills and valleys with lush green grass.

When a beloved pet dies, the pet goes to this place. There is always food and water and warm spring weather. The old and frail animals are young again. Those who are maimed are made whole again. They play all day with each other.

There is only one thing missing. They are not with their special person who loved them on Earth. So each day they run and play until the day comes when one suddenly stops playing and looks up! The nose twitches! The ears are up! The eyes are staring! And this one suddenly runs from the group.

You have been seen, and when you and your special friend meet, you take him or her in your arms and embrace. Your face is kissed again and again, and you look once more into the eyes of your trusting pet.

Then you cross the Rainbow Bridge together, never again to be separated.

Note: This version of *The Rainbow Bridge* was provided in the pets section of America Online. It was also used in a "Dear Abby" column several years ago. (Unattributed.)

# Contents

ix

# *Introduction*

You've recently lost your much-loved dog, who always bounded up to meet you when you came home after a long, hard day, with unconditional acceptance and joy. He has died and you miss him terribly. Or maybe it was your cherished cat who has died, the beautiful feline you and your children carefully chose together over a decade ago. She's gone now and you can scarcely believe it.

It could be a rabbit, a gerbil, horse, bird, turtle, squirrel, or any type of a wide variety of pets that you care for and love. And now this animal has died. The common denominator is the love—and the loss.

You feel so very sad, maybe even devastated. So what do you do? If you're like most people, you shed your tears behind closed doors, in secret, and don't tell anyone outside your family how you feel. You think that maybe you can effectively contain it in a little corner of your mind. You may not even tell other family members about the emotions you're struggling with.

You perceive that they might think you're silly, or that you're overreacting. But they might also be going through exactly the same turmoil—and *they're* not telling *you* because they fear that you might think that they're silly or overreacting.

You probably don't tell anyone at work. And take some time off? Come on. Soldier on. Time off from work is for "real problems," like a death in your family. Only maybe your pet was part of your family, to you.

If you're a man, it might be even harder to talk about your grief. Because "real men" don't cry, certainly not about pets that die. Real men don't grieve very long either. They especially don't get broken up over an animal, right? Wrong! But that's the popular perception.

Tom, a retired man and avid animal lover, said he told other men at the gym where he works out that he was upset about the rapidly failing health of Peepers, his pet squirrel. He said he was very distressed about the prospect of euthanasia. But Tom didn't meet with positive feedback at all. These reactions made his emotional pain worse. He stopped talking about his feelings with his friends. He kept it inside. Nobody wants to be seen as a wimp or to be publicly ridiculed.

This book is for you if you are grieving over the loss of an animal companion. This book is to tell you that it is okay, indeed normal, to feel sad. Not all pet owners grieve deeply, but many do. If you're reading this right now, you're one of them. But you'll find it's also possible to work through your grief. Not around it—you really can't skirt it or ignore it. But there are tactics and strategies you can use to cope with your grief and to help your children and others cope. Some good coping ideas are included within these pages.

Why this book and why now? Because many people don't understand grief over a dying or deceased pet, and in our high-tech world, it may seem strange to stop long enough to cry over a pet lost to you. What too many people don't realize is that grief for a dead or dying companion animal *is* normal and that many people—men, women, and children of all ages—grieve when their companion animals die.

There are people of all sexes and age groups who are devoted to their pets and grieve very deeply upon their death. Over half of the grieving pet owners I interviewed were men who were very devoted to their pets and very distressed when their companion animals died.

In one study, middle-aged pet owners whose animals had died were asked to rate the stress level of the animal's death as well as the stress level of other difficult experiences such as divorce, losing a job, and so on.

What the researchers learned was that the pet's death was the one traumatic experience most frequently experienced by the respondents. The participants said that the death of their pet was not as stressful as the death of someone in their immediate family, but it was *more* stressful than the death of relatives not living with them. Twenty-eight percent of the husbands and 48 percent of the wives said that the death of their companion animal was either "extremely" or "quite" disturbing. It's clear from this study and others, as well as plenty of anecdotal evidence, that the death of a pet is often very difficult for the human owner.

Yet there are still many people who can't comprehend the grief you feel. After all, it was *only* a dog. It was *only* a cat. Or *only* a lizard. Even if they are sympathetic, they may say, hey, go get another one, not realizing that a longtime companion animal is more difficult than that to replace. They just don't understand that pets are not interchangeable commodities. And that you are grieving over a very particular pet—the one that was special and unique to you, and that was like a family member or a friend to you.

In fact, many pet owners have stated that they receive more in the form of friendship and companionship from their pets than they do from their neighbors or friends. In a 1984 *Psychology Today* survey of thirteen thousand people, an amazing 80 percent of the respondents expressed such a sentiment—that they gained more friendship and companionship from their animals. Sometimes people say that they have grieved the loss of a companion animal more than the loss of a parent or friend—this feeling is fairly common, although many people don't express such emotions openly, for fear of social disapproval.

Part of the problem is that we just don't like to think about death at all, especially when it concerns those who are close to us. For example, in 1995, cartoonist Lynn Johnston ran a column in her strip, *For Better or for Worse,* in which Farley, the cartoon dog, died. Her newspaper syndicate immediately received numerous phone calls complaining about the dog's death. Apparently, the dog should have lived forever. People even wrote letters to the editors of newspapers, stating their sorrow at the "death" of Farley and how much they would miss him.

But as Johnston "grew" her characters older in the comic strip, she said she also had resolved that the dog would age too. Thus, she made this choice to have him die. Her cartoon dog saved a child from a raging river and then died, a hero, of a heart attack. The characters in the strip mourned and the child who was saved was comforted by her father when she blamed herself for the dog's death.

But this sort of realistic and positive treatment of an animal's death is highly unusual in the media. It's not that it was shocking—we as a culture are nearly inured to violence. We see rapes, murders, and all sorts of real-life violence in newspapers and on television. But rarely is the death of a companion animal addressed at all, despite the fact that it's an event that affects so many people so profoundly. The death of an animal hurts, on an up-close and personal level.

There is good news on the horizon—increasing recognition that losing a companion animal hurts. In fact, there is a lot of hope for bereaved pet owners because people *are* starting to talk about their sorrow. Support groups are springing up. Veterinarians are starting to receive special training in understanding the grief of pet loss. Scientists are beginning studies and surveys on the human-animal bond, a linkage that has lasted for thousands of years.

In increasing numbers of cases, professors are seeing pet death as a way to explain the concept of bereavement to students. Dr. Kenneth Curl, a professor at the University of Central Oklahoma in Oklahoma City, offers graduate and undergraduate courses on death and dying. Integrated with his course is information on pet grief, which he feels is an important addition to the curriculum.

Curl says that on "Career Days" at local schools, his students talk to children about pets that have died and the children gain a great deal from this experience. "They always get invited back," Curl says of his students. He also notes that sometimes in his course, his students acknowledge and accept a grief they've had themselves over pets that died in the past—sometimes acknowledging their losses for the very first time.

All of these changes are healthy for people who are grieving the loss of a companion animal because it's important to realize that it's okay to be sad when your pet dies. It will hurt. And it will eventually get better.

These are the basic messages of this book, based on interviews with pet owners and counselors nationwide. They want you to know that grief over the death of your pet is natural and it's normal. They want you to know there are things you can do to make it better for yourself and your family. They want you to learn from their mistakes and their successes.

*When Your Pet Dies* is about acknowledging and accepting that sadness and coping with it. It's about giving yourself permission to grieve. In addition, it's about learning to help others cope with their own grief, whether it's an elderly parent or a child who needs special attention. It's about learning not to make the too common mistake of ignoring the grief or trying to cheer people up.

Although the majority of people who own pets have cats or dogs or rabbits, horses, and other "mainstream" animals, it is also true that the companion animals for many people are lizards, snakes, pigs, and a wide variety of other pets that may be considered unusual or "exotic."

Sometimes pet owners of a lizard or a hamster may feel even more "disenfranchised" about their grieving than a cat or dog owner—feeling even more strongly that they're not allowed to be upset. Why? Because more people can relate to loving a cat or dog (although they may not understand the profundity of grief at its loss) but may not "get it" that people can love other unusual pets just as much. I have tried to include examples and anecdotes of a wide variety of pet owners and the pets who they love.

In reading *When Your Pet Dies*, you may wish to skip immediately to the chapters that you feel are relevant to your situation; for example, if your pet died suddenly, you may wish to read this chapter first and ignore others. I recommend you at least skim all the chapters, because anecdotes and advice in another chapter may provide you with insight and comfort you need.

Although I don't want to go overboard being "politically correct," I have tried to use nonoffensive terminology. For example, some animal lovers prefer the term "companion animal" or "animal companion" to "pet." The people I interviewed used both terms and so am I. To me, a pet is an animal that one loves and cares for and who also fulfills a companionship role.

The word "owner," although technically correct, can seem cold when referring to the positive and loving relationship that humans have with their pets. So I have tried to vary "owner" with "caretaker" or sometimes merely "human." The truth is, however, that legally we do own our pets, no matter how much we do love them and see them as family members. Others have expressed favoring the words "steward" or "guardian," in reference to the person caring for the animal, but those terms don't seem accurate or very descriptive to me.

Of course, it's important to note that most pet owners don't see their animal as a "pet" or "companion animal''; instead the animal is ''Prince'' or ''Amelia'' or whatever. The relationship is very personal to them.

It's undeniably true that most pet caretakers love their pets very much, and sometimes are closer with them than they are with human companions. I fully acknowledge this deep love for animals and can attest to this fact through the many poignant interviews I've had with bereaved pet caretakers.

I hope that this book will help you and your loved ones deal with the death of your pets. I know that I can't take away your pain, but what I can do is offer tactics and strategies and some basic everyday tips that have helped others and may help you too.

# 1

## *How We Relate to Pets*

Throughout our existence on earth, pets have been used for hunting, protection, and for companionship.

In 1978, a tomb was uncovered in northern Israel that held the remains of a human and a dog who were buried together—about twelve thousand years ago. The hand of the deceased person was placed on the animal's shoulder, clearly indicating the care that someone knew that person had for his animal. Scientific evidence shows that dogs were domesticated about twelve thousand years ago, cats about six thousand years ago. Archaeologist Stewart Schrever discovered what is considered to be the oldest pet cemetery, dating back to 6500 B.C., which means people have loved pets enough to memorialize them for nearly 8,500 years. (And probably a lot longer.)

Cats fell out of favor during the Middle Ages, when people identified them with witchcraft. Too bad! Had there been more cats, they might have aborted the scourge of the bubonic plague, spread by rats. People have regained their senses and now cats account for the majority of pets in the United States.

Perhaps the current era is an especially good time to love a pet. Why? Because most of us are separated geographically from our parents and relatives and the people we grew up with. And it can be a very big cold world out there. Sometimes you can feel like you are just a number. Or maybe a lot of numbers. You are your phone number, your Social Security number, your ATM number, your credit-card number, your patient account number, and undoubtedly many more. You may sometimes feel diminished and unimportant.

But not to your pet—this animal sees you as wonderful, great, even godlike! Your companion animal has no mental yardstick for continually evaluating your performance. Sure, he can be happy or sad—but not critical of you.

No mere number to your companion animal, you are instead the person who feeds and shelters and loves him, and he returns your love over and over, unconditionally. The most devoted human mother could not offer such unconditional love. In addition, pets don't require a lot of talk (or any!) or explanations about why you did or did not do something. Pets remain at your side, silently and companionably. They need you. They accept you. They love you.

Your pet also loves you no matter how much money you make and whether you're on the fast track to success or on unemployment compensation. It doesn't matter at all to your pet, the love is still there.

Time is another factor/problem in today's hectic world—it seems to get eaten up very fast. Even with so many timesaving devices, time often seems just to slip by as you rush around from one task to the next. Yet companion animals may force you to pay attention to them, and by doing so, you take notice of the world around you. And, hopefully, you celebrate that you are alive!

Animals will accept a quick fix of your quality time or a bit of affection. They'll take as much as you can give. And when they die, you miss this unconditional love and affection.

## Time to Grieve

In our hurry-up world where we can bank and eat on the run while intermittently talking on car telephones, it's expected that most problems should be resolved quickly and efficiently. After all, if I can receive a fax from Russia and talk to people across the United States in one day, then why couldn't I—or you—deal quickly with most other problems?

The reason is that when you form a deep attachment to an animal or to a person, it's not so readily given up. I think that people sometimes assume the hyperspeed of our lifestyles and our communication styles can be applied to the much slower process of emotional health and healing.

You can't slap a Band-Aid on your sadness or have quickie surgery to fix it in your local hospital. It just doesn't work that way when it comes to emotional healing. Nor can you realistically limit your grieving to an hour or a day—it can't be programmed. But there are ways to help you with the grieving process, and this book provides some suggestions and strategies.

## GENERAL REASONS WHY PEOPLE BECOME PET CARETAKERS

Researchers have recently begun taking very hard looks at why people own pets. One obvious motivation is that they love animals. In addition, if they have children, they want to teach their children to care for and love animals too—as their parents taught them when they were children. Or they may want a pet to be a companion to themselves, in either a "friend" role or a "child" role.

Caring for an animal can give a child a feeling of competency and responsibility. Children also enjoy the unconditional love and acceptance they receive from their pets.

Being aware of these various roles can help us understand why pets are so important to us in life and why we are so saddened by their deaths.


## Pets Have Personalities

Animal lovers know their pets as very unique and special, and often brag about their qualities. I am guilty of this myself. My husband and I have taught our cats to "speak" and to "roll over" on command and I think they are unusually bright animals. Many other human companions also speak of their pets as exceptional and special beings.

I also know my two cats have very distinctive personalities. One is very shy and the other is far more aggressive. One is talkative and the other rarely speaks. And so on. Every animal is different and unique, and is special to its human companion.

As a result, when a much-loved animal with these special qualities dies, it is the loss of the uniqueness of the animal that is mourned.

## Animals Can Serve as Stress Buffers

Companion animals have been known to act as a stress buffer for people whose human companions are seriously ill or have died. According to a study done by the U.S. Army Veterinary Corps of more than nine hundred pet owners, over half of the respondents said that their pets were important to them during periods of crisis, illness, relocations, or the temporary absence of a spouse and depression.

The mere presence of a pet during difficult times can help people "get through." As a result, when the pet dies, the person may feel at a loss, knowing that the companion animal that has been there in good times and really bad times is now gone forever, and will no longer be able to provide that loving support.

## Health Benefits to Pet Ownership

Pets can also improve your health. The list below cites a few health advantages.

Lower blood pressure
Lower cholesterol rate
Lower triglyceride rate
Faster recovery from hospitalization
Improved concentration
Weight loss
Improved attitude

A pet can also reduce stress and anxiety in a child. In a study of twenty-six children with an average age of twelve years, researchers found that blood pressure was reduced significantly when a dog was in the room compared with when the dog was not in the room. A study of abused children revealed that they were more likely than nonabused children to seek love and affection from their pets and to use them as confidants.

Unfortunately, it is also true that pets are more likely to be victimized by someone in the abusive household, possibly the person who abused the child. And if the child has been abused extremely, it may be the child who hurts the animal. Some institutions that care for emotionally disturbed children provide pets under supervision to the children, which can be a very rewarding and safe experience for both animal and child.

Elderly people in nursing homes and autistic children in institutions are two more groups that have showed very positive gains when pets are brought into their environments. Some prison systems have brought in animals for the inmates and were amazed at the positive way the pets were received.

## THE ROLE OF PETS

People interact with and relate to their companion animals in very different ways. Some people treat their pets as a family member. The pet sleeps with them, goes on trips with them, and generally shares their lives. Said one pet owner who considers his pets part of his family, "Dogs repay our care with total devotion. I don't care where they are on the evolutionary chain. Seeing that love and devotion will cause great grief when the animal dies."

Some pet caretakers treat their pets like children and

enjoy caring for them and babying them. In fact, some pet owners have reported a new love interest not liking the pet and saying, "It's him or me." And if the pet hater didn't relent? The pet stayed.

In one unusual case reported in *People* magazine, Martin Scot Kosins, a concert pianist, quit his job and devoted a year of his life to his dying dog. He later authored the book *Maya's First Rose*.

When they perceive their animals as childlike, pet caretakers may celebrate the pet's birthday with some special food and a present. (We celebrate our cats' birthdays in our family. We eat cake and the birthday cat shares tuna with her sister.) In one study of pet owners, researchers found that some pet caretakers talk to their animals as if they were infants, in a higher voice and a slower cadence than normal speech. In addition, the pet owners' faces relax while talking to the animal companion. In one case, a woman whose dog died was very grief-stricken and people she knew just couldn't understand this because she had three other dogs. But the dog who died was the only female, and she related to that dog as a child.

Many pet owners believe that they can effectively communicate with their companion animals. It's also true that the majority of pet owners talk to their pets. In a study performed by the U.S. Army, 77 percent perceived that their pets understood what they were saying to them and 74 percent felt that their companion animal responded to their communications. Fifty-nine percent also said that the animal was responsive to their changing moods. If they were happy, the animal responded in a positive way. If they were angry or upset, the animal might cringe or hide. (In some cases, the pet tried to act as a peacemaker by attracting attention to himself.) In another study, a third of pet owners said they used their pets as confidants.

## Pets as Siblings

Sometimes animals are even seen as a sort of sibling to a human child, if the primary caretaker is a parent. In fact, there can be some "sibling rivalry" if the parents pay too much attention to the pet. One college student complained that when he came home from school, the dog got the good leftovers, not him. He was mildly aggrieved but laughed about it.

Pets can be extremely important to children, and many children enjoy the companionship and playfulness of their pets. Playing with the pet also allows the child to get rid of any excess energy.

## Pets as Recreational Companions

Sometimes an animal companion is important because it can engage in physical activities with you—play ball, hunt, even drag you out of your old easy chair when it's time to take her for a walk.

Often when a pet dies, for some time afterward pet caretakers report that they automatically reach for the pet's leash at the regular walk time or they unthinkingly listen for the animal's familiar noises. Then they remember and feel sad and possibly even a little silly. These are normal reactions of grieving pet owners.

## Pets as Projections of Yourself

In some cases, the pet owner strongly identifies with the features and personality of an animal companion, either as the owner perceives him or herself to be or wants to be. For this reason, a young man who chooses a virile and healthy male dog may be loath to have the animal neutered.

A study of dog owners looked at the Great Dane and found that this breed of dog served as a symbol of the owner's masculinity, virility, and strength, whereas a Chihuahua was often perceived as symbolic of feminine characteristics. Thus the very macho man is far more likely to own a Great Dane or other strong dog than he is to own a small dog. (It's unclear how women feel about all of this; for example, women may own large dogs for protection and security, rather than to make a statement of invulnerability or strength.)

If you see your pet as an extension of yourself, then the pet's death can be very traumatic and you may feel like a part of you died too.

## Pets as Cotherapists

Increasing numbers of nursing homes and other institutions use pets to help people. Virginia Miller, a counselor in private practice in Oklahoma City, told me that she uses pets to help children who are clients. "They'll talk to the dogs when they won't talk to me," she says. She says that her animals love all people.

Some experts have suggested that a pet serves as a sort of "transitional object" to adulthood, similar to the teddy bear or blanket of the preschooler. In this respect, the pet may be very helpful to adolescents. No self-respecting teenager can get away with carrying around a beat-up old teddy bear or a torn blanket loved since infancy—but they can hug and pay lots of attention to their companion animal.

## People in the Same Family Have Different Relationships with Pets

If you have more than one person in your household, then there is probably more than one human-animal relationship going on. One person may baby the pet, another may take the pet for runs and exercise, and a third may ignore the animal altogether. In turn, the pet will relate to the humans in different ways, attracted more to some than to others.

As a result, when a pet dies, the intensity of grief and the way that grief is exhibited varies among family members. Some will openly grieve. Others will care deeply but will try to hide or repress their feelings. And others will be sad but not grieve deeply. Even family members who didn't like the pet will be affected.

## Yet Pet Grief Is Hard for People to Understand

With all the many reasons for becoming very attached to your companion animals, why is it that many people just don't understand, or say that they don't understand, why a person would mourn for a pet that has died? I think that this lack of compassion could be in part because the person has never had a pet or doesn't feel deeply about pets. It's not necessarily that they are uncaring or mean people. They truly just don't "get it." No matter how hard you try to explain, you probably will be unsuccessful.

So when people press us to "get on" with our lives, grow up, deal with it, maybe instead we should realize that there are aspects of life that scare or distress us all. You're upset that you lost a pet—the person who doesn't understand might be devastated if his computer broke!

Don't waste your time trying to convey your feelings to people who are baffled by them. Instead, talk to other animal lovers, who can give you the empathy and support you need. Try not to take offense and realize that in many cases, people are thoughtlessly tossing off comments, not trying to send a verbal arrow through your heart.

## Disenfranchised Grief

Experts also view pet death as a kind of disenfranchised (or not accepted by others) grief. A woman who has always longed for a child and who has had a miscarriage can be one example of this. Or the man who has lost his job, which made up a major part of his identity—he's frightened, upset, and grief-stricken about his loss.

The pet caretaker whose pet dies also suffers disenfranchised grief when people say to them, "It was *only* a lizard."—or rabbit, duck, cat, dog, and so forth. Says Myrna Sogalnick, who leads a bereavement support group at the University of Wisconsin, "You could go into work tomorrow and you could say to your boss, 'My fifth cousin ten times removed died over the weekend and we were really close. I need to take a couple of days off.' And chances are the boss wouldn't blink. But if you go into work and say, 'My dog died over the weekend and we were very close. I need some time off,' you'll probably get a very different response. People trivialize the loss of a companion animal.''

The next chapter discusses the nature of grief and how different people may express it. We'll also talk about some ways you can cope with this grief.

# 2

# *People Grieve Differently*

Because of the many different personalities, ages, and interests of pet lovers, when a companion animal dies, methods of grieving and the intensity of that grief may vary considerably. Nor can one always tell how people feel by merely looking at their faces, because some people are very adept at hiding their emotions. It's also important to note that children often grieve very differently from adults.

There is no one way of grieving your loss that is "right" or "wrong," and it's important for family members to understand that. The person who suffers in silence may resent the person who cries publicly, seeing her or him as hysterical, while the person who is openly upset may see the quietly grieving person as uncaring.

It's important to understand that not only do people have different depths of feelings, but they also have different ways of dealing with those feelings. Acceptance of your own feelings, whatever they are, and acceptance of the feelings of others, will help the entire family unit. It is very unreasonable and unrealistic to expect everyone in your family to feel just as you do. They can't.

## When a Pet Dies, the Family Balance Shifts

However it is that we relate to our companion animals, when the pet dies, things change. Even people who say they are not that attached to pets become sad. Things are different, patterns are broken.

If the pet was a direct or indirect focus for family discussions or concerns, that focus is gone. The family needs to redirect itself to new goals—which may, eventually, include acquiring a new pet.

## Even Caring Others Can Make It Worse

Because many people in our culture are uncomfortable with a display of emotions, particularly serious grief, even those people who care about you and who are fellow animal lovers might try to "talk you out" of your grief.

Here are some common tactics they may try:

• Why don't you go on a vacation and get your mind off things?
• Maybe you need to take Prozac or some other antidepressant.
• You should get another (dog, cat, etc.).
• Why don't you take on some new projects and keep yourself busy so you don't think about this?
• Now, I know you're going to just snap right out of this. You have to stop dwelling on the past.

These comments don't help—but keep in mind that most people are trying, albeit ineffectually, to comfort or distract you. They want you to feel better, and don't understand that their words can't achieve that goal.

## Intensity of Grief

Scientists have actually studied and compared grief among pet caretakers who have lost a pet, in order to find out if there are some types of people who grieve more than others.

For example, in one study, researchers found that grief levels were directly affected by the level of attachment of the caretaker with the animal, the suddenness of the animal's death, and whether or not the person lived alone.

The caretaker's level of attachment was determined by the names people called their pets; for example, a high level of attachment was assumed if the person said their pet was "everything," "baby," or "child," while a low bonding rating was assigned if the primary way the person regarded a pet was as a "protector." As expected, the intensity of grief was directly associated with the level of attachment the person felt to a pet.

Other researchers have found that when the pet has been very ill and received special care from the owner, the grief at the death of the pet is accentuated.

This is understandable for two reasons. First, the person who takes special care of a companion animal is probably already very attached to the pet. Second, by virtue of providing caregiving, the attachment can deepen even further, making the loss of the pet very painful.

Frank, a physician and pet lover, was on a camping trip when it became extremely cold and he could see that his beagle, Charger, was actually in danger of dying. He took the dog into his sleeping bag with him all night and his body warmth enabled Charger to survive. This experience bonded the man and dog and they were thereafter inseparable. When Charger died, the man was devastated.

Said Cathy of her cat, Spot, "I was absolutely grief-stricken, and I have to say that this was the most important loss in my life. His death saddened me more than even my parents' deaths. This cat brought me back from a very hard time in my life and gave me reason to live at one point. His suddenly being gone just seemed unbelievable and insurmountable."

She did, however, get beyond this pain and wants others to know that it does get easier to bear over time. "There are moments when you think you'll never be normal again, but time corrects that eventually. There will be a time when the sad memories are replaced by ones that make you smile and brighten your days."

Some pet caretakers say they were drawn to their pets who hated everyone else but them, thus singling out the pet owner as a special person worthy of affection. It is hard to deal with the death in that case because that special bond has been destroyed. In some cases the animal itself was very unattractive and rather ill-tempered, and owners said no one else would ever have loved this animal. But they did.

Grief may be manifested in many different ways, a grieving person passes through many stages and emotions. This is the subject of the next chapter.

# 3

## Stages of Grief

Just as you do after the death of a beloved person, you may experience different phases of your grief when your companion animal dies. Elisabeth Kübler-Ross long ago attempted to explain these stages, and others have expanded or redefined her explanations. I'll discuss here the key phases that humans may go through when a pet dies. Keep in mind that you may go through all or only some of these.

### Denial

Denial is a very common first stage. This terrible thing could not have happened—it's not possible. There may be a feeling of shock, numbness, and unreality. One veterinarian reported that after telling a person that her animal was terminally ill, the pet owner kept insisting that the baffled vet trim her cat's claws. The woman was not ready to deal with the inevitable, and was revealing her denial very clearly.

Denial isn't necessarily a bad thing—it's one way we humans have of initially coping with severe problems until we have a chance to prepare ourselves emotionally and intellectually. It's when we never—or for a very prolonged period—accept the reality of a situation that it becomes problematic.

A complicating factor can be that the caretaker just never really thought about the death of a pet, and seemed to think that the pet would live forever. When it doesn't, this comes as a severe shock. It wasn't really that they thought the pet was immortal. It just was presumed that the pet would always be there, as a sort of "given."

## Bargaining

Another grieving stage is "bargaining." This stage usually occurs if the animal is seriously ill but hasn't yet died. The caretaker may try to bargain with God or promise to himself that he will always and forever be good if only the pet will continue to live. She will buy only the best pet food. She will pay lots more attention to the animal.

## Anger

Anger is another phase that grieving caretakers may pass through. You may be unreasonably angry at a family member or wish to blame someone. Some people blame the veterinarian, often unfairly. He or she *should* be able to heal your animal and *should* be able to prevent death. They do try, but cannot always succeed. Said Janine after the loss of her ferret Frankie, "My husband was violently angry. He pounded the side of our van with fists after we lost him and he cried. He also made idle threats against the vet, was unspeakably moody with me for days, and was sulky at work."

Sometimes people get angry with God. "It's okay to get mad at God," says Virginia Miller, a pet bereavement counselor. "Nobody says you can't get angry with the landlord!" But understand that death is an inevitable part of life, and should be accepted as such.

Anger is often turned inward and transformed into guilt, as you think of the multitudes of things you "should" have done. Many people will take self-blame to an almost unbelievable level, at least as an initial reaction to the sad news. In some cases, you may even be angry at the pet itself, for running in front of a car, for example, although you yelled at him about a hundred times before to not do that. You are also angry at the pet for leaving you.

### Acceptance

When acceptance of what has happened occurs, the person may still feel profoundly distressed—"acceptance" doesn't necessarily mean you're okay with this loss. Instead, it means that you accept that your pet is really truly gone, but you are still heartsick about it. This is a very difficult stage to work through. Talking to sympathetic others can help—you may wish to join a pet bereavement support group. (See Chapter Four.)

### Resolution

The last stage of the grieving process is the resolution phase, when you can bear the thought of your loss. You are still unhappy about it, but you can focus more on the good times you and your pet shared together. Said one animal lover, "I'm starting to get to the point where

I can laugh about the funny things she once did—and there were many of them!''

Many people are very ambivalent about their feelings during the entire grieving process. They are drawn toward the lost pet and at the same time they realize they must accept reality and know that the pet is truly gone. As a result, within their minds they careen back and forth from past memories to the present reality.

It's important to note that these phases are not orderly and consecutive. You may skip some of them altogether and may also revert back and forth between them. Describing these stages of grief is one way to understand what many people go through in a normal grieving process.

## SYMPTOMS AND EXPRESSIONS OF GRIEF

What surprises, and sometimes distresses or baffles, a lot of people is that many of the emotions they feel when a valued person dies are the same emotions they feel when a beloved companion animal dies. ''I think people go through exactly the same thing as they do in the death of a parent or a sibling, based on what I've seen in my office,'' says Barry Schwartz, MD, a psychiatrist in Bala Cynwyd, Pennsylvania.

He says it's also important to differentiate grief from depression. They may feel very much alike—but they're different. ''With depression, you feel the world outside is okay but there's something wrong or sick or bad inside you,'' says Schwartz. You may feel the world might be better off without you. (Please note that sometimes grieving pet owners do become severely depressed and should seek professional help if that happens. See the section later in this chapter which will help you gauge whether you are experiencing a major depression.)

Conversely, grief is a deep sadness and has to do with a loss from outside. It doesn't necessarily mean you are bad—although it does mean that you feel bad.

Many people cry over their loss and veterinarians say that men, too, may cry like babies. Caretakers may also find themselves preoccupied with thoughts of the pet after the death and find themselves drawn to objects and toys that were familiar to the animal. Sounds may remind the person of the pet. Smells may remind them too—the smell of the pet may still be on a favorite blanket or object. (And you should be careful about immediately throwing out every item associated with or used by the pet—keeping a few items for a while can help ease your pain.)

## Guilt and Self-Blame Are Very Common

As mentioned earlier, you may also be guilt-ridden with the "what-ifs" or "if onlys." If only you had locked the cat from the porch, where she never went anyway, then in that split second when you turned your back, your cat wouldn't have been able to kill your pet lizard while it was sunning itself. And on and on.

The guilt may be very irrational, and if you think about it, you know, intellectually, that it is. And yet you still ruminate. If only you had not taken the dog to be groomed, she would not have gotten sick. Or if only you had remembered to give your pet that pill three weeks before she died, maybe she wouldn't have become ill.

Hopefully, your veterinarian, family friends, and others will remind you of all the loving care you provided your animal, maybe for many years. Listen to them! And try to forgive yourself for any petty errors you may have made.

This is hard. Because, basically, no matter what you did do, you will probably wonder what you "should" have done. One counselor said if the animal dies at home, the owner thinks he or she should have brought the pet to the animal hospital. And if the animal dies in the animal hospital, the owner thinks the pet should have died at home.

Don't search for reasons to blame yourself, and don't listen to others who want to assign blame. Certainly it is most unhelpful to second-guess and criticize past actions which cannot be changed. It's unlikely that the person hasn't already thought of every contingency that he or she "could" or "should" have done, and thus they have beat on themselves quite enough already!

One way you might combat the self-blaming tendency is to imagine that your friend had a pet and it died in similar circumstances to your own pet. Now, do you think your friend should be blamed and criticized? Probably not. So try to stop blaming yourself.

You might also feel as if when the pet died, a part of you died too. This is because of the many experiences you shared with the animal and the bond that has built up, often over many years. "I've had a terrible time coming to terms with this loss," says Tina, owner of Merlin, an eight-year-old boxer that was recently euthanized. "It's been a month and I've had a difficult time sleeping and eating and I've lost weight."

## Studies of Expressions of Grief

The Veterinary Hospital of the University of Pennsylvania has established a social-work service for pet owners whose pets have died. In 1983, their researchers studied 218 pet owners who had been referred to the service. Reasons for referrals ranged from the owners' difficulties related to euthanizing their pets to the owners' distress over the death of, or diagnosis of a serious illness in, a companion animal.

Of the subjects studied, 93 percent found their daily lives had been disrupted and their sleeping and eating patterns altered. They ate more or less than usual and had difficulty sleeping and/or experienced nightmares. For about 70 percent, social activities decreased, and they stayed at home more and mingled with people far less than was normal for them. About 45 percent reported missing between one to three days of work, generally taking sick days or vacation days. Social workers found that a major problem for the pet owners was the perceived lack of support from their friends, relatives, and colleagues.

## Physical Symptoms

You may have respiratory complaints such as shortness of breath or hyperventilation (rapid breathing). Barry told me that within hours after Blue's death, he arrived home from the veterinarian's office and started hyperventilating. He was afraid he would fall, so he lay down on the kitchen floor until the feeling had passed.

Some people have gastrointestinal difficulties and get

stomachaches or diarrhea. If you have any or all of these symptoms, you should seek medical attention. Sometimes a loss can actually make a person physically sick or make them more likely to become ill and it's important to verify with your doctor what is going on.

Symptoms include:

Crying or sobbing
Diarrhea or constipation
Inability to eat or overeating
Light-headedness
Shortness of breath
Sleep disorder
Extreme tiredness
Stomach pains

## Mental-Health Difficulties

Your emotional health may be greatly affected by the death of your companion animal. You may feel extremely lonely. You may feel restless and unable to sit still, but you don't really know what to do. Sometimes people think over and over about the circumstances of the pet's death, seeking for something that could have been done differently. You may also feel disorganized and confused; for example, you may find it impossible to finish a task before your mind wanders off.

Some bereaved pet owners believe they are actually losing their sanity, particularly if they have never faced a major loss or grieving situation in the past. Rarely are these fears justified. It's just that because generally we don't talk about pet grief in our society, people have no emotional yardstick to evaluate themselves against.

You may find yourself unconsciously searching for the animal. "I still keep looking for Merlin," said Tina of her boxer. "He was always my dog, always just about attached to my side. I miss always tripping over Merlin because he had to be as close to me as possible in whatever room I was in." Some owners have stated that they unconsciously try to avoid stepping on the absent pet.

You may even imagine that you see or hear your animal—you have not lost your mind if this happens a few times. It's a common grief reaction.

Psychological reactions include:

Confusion
Helplessness
Anxiety
Panic
Fear
Shock
Sadness
Grief
Hallucinations related to the animal ("seeing" the animal, even though you know it has died).
Drop in self-esteem
Guilt
Numbness
Confusion

You may experience some, all, or none of these. Every person grieves differently. The death of a favorite pet can bring back memories of other pets that were loved and lost, even memories of other people who were dear to the individual. If your pet died of cancer, it may bring to mind family members who have also died of cancer. Or it may bring up unrelated but unhappy events from the past.

## Fear of Grief

Because grieving for an animal that has died is generally not socially acceptable, a person who finds himself sobbing and repeatedly thinking about the animal may wonder if he's normal.

Although some people do grieve very excessively, most people's grief can be considered "normal." Sometimes the person will burst into tears for no apparent reason weeks after the death. This behavior is within the normal range. But sometimes the grief can increase to an extent that a person really needs to seek professional counseling, particularly if she has had other recent losses. All the losses taken together may seem too much to deal with.

If someone is neglecting their personal hygiene for weeks, and has virtually lost their appetite and can no longer enjoy former activities, even at a reduced level, then this person may have fallen into a "major" or clinical depression.

The good news is that, in most cases, depression is treatable. The person needs to talk about this loss and receive validation and acknowledgment, whether through a pet bereavement counselor or support group or through a mental-health professional. (See Chapter Four for more information on such counselors and groups.)

## Stuck in Grief

In some cases, people become terribly distraught and cannot seem to overcome their grief. Sometimes the grief may be tied in with other losses. For example, one woman who was completely bereft needed professional counseling. What the counselor learned was that this woman's daughter had died six months before her dog. The dog was the woman's last "tie" to her daughter, and when it was gone, the woman fell to pieces.

In another case, a child became terribly upset weeks after a pet's death and her parents consulted a mental-health professional. The parents had not been seriously grief-stricken by their dog's death and thought their child felt the same way. They then learned that the child had gotten the idea that if her parents didn't much care when the dog died, they probably wouldn't really care if she died too.

Upon discovering this, the parents assured her that they loved her very deeply and would be devastated if she died. The girl and her parents learned of the profound and complex aspects of grief and how it affects people differently.

## Severely Bereaved People

Although people of all ages and circumstances could become seriously depressed by the loss of a pet, there are commonalities among distressed people referred to social workers and counselors.

The age of the pet at death and the length of the relationship between animal companion and human is very significant. Generally, the longer the animal has been in your life, the more difficult it will be to accept his death. Another key factor is whether or not the human caretaker has suffered the loss of a loved person within the past two years. The death of your pet can be seen as one loss piled upon others.

When the person who died was associated in some way with your pet that died, this can intensify your grieving. For example, if the disease that the animal died from had also been suffered by the human caretaker, this makes the loss more difficult.

A very significant factor related to bereavement is that a person often associates the animal with an extremely positive or extremely negative event. For example, the pet could have been given to the owner as a gift by a husband or wife. Or the pet could have saved the human from death or injury.

In the next chapter, we will talk about ways people effectively deal with their grief.

# 4

## *Coping with Your Grief*

The ancient Egyptians showed their grief at the loss of a family cat by shaving off their eyebrows. And if it was a dog that died, they shaved their entire bodies! Maybe the Egyptians had the right idea in one sense: they acknowledged the sadness that accompanies the loss of a beloved animal. You don't have to go quite so far, but one thing you do need to do is acknowledge your grief and accept it as a valid emotion. This chapter offers suggestions for yourself and other family members for making it through the grief period. There are some times of the year when losing your pet can be especially traumatic; for example, during holiday seasons. And there are instances when the grief comes back to you all over again, such as your pet's birthday or even your own birthday. These issues are also covered in this chapter.

## Do Veterinarians Always Know How to Comfort You?

Readers can probably answer this question themselves. Most veterinarians are very caring and compassionate people, yet they may feel at a loss in dealing with the profound sorrow of a bereaved pet owner. Remember that your vet is human and may or may not be good at comforting you.

Increasing numbers of veterinary schools are offering training on pet loss to veterinarians, and according to Laurel Lagoni, codirector of the Changes program at the Colorado State University Veterinary Teaching Hospital in Fort Collins, her veterinarian students receive extensive training in this area.

It's likely that future generations of veterinarians nationwide will be very sensitized to this issue. But this doesn't mean your forty-something vet is hard-hearted! Many older and experienced vets have learned through experience how to console bereaved pet owners.

### SOME DO'S AND DON'TS

Based on the experiences of others who have mourned the loss of your companion animal, here are a few basic do's and don'ts related to your immediate pet loss.

### It's Okay to Be Sad

One point that is impressed in this book over and over is that you can expect to feel a wide variety of emotions when your companion animal dies, but the primary one will be deep sadness. So profound an emotion can be scary and it can be disturbing to lose control over your emotions. Accept that you are a human animal and that you will be sad and this is normal. Eventually you will feel better and will look back and remember the good times with your animal companion.

## Find Someone to Talk to

Okay, maybe the people you work with or your best friend think you're being just plain silly to be so sad over a pet's death. Find someone who can understand, whether that person is a friend in your circle, someone on an on-line computer service, someone in a local pet grief support group, or elsewhere. Seek and you shall find someone.

## Don't Make Any Major Decisions

When you are upset about your pet's death, it is not a good time to quit your job, move to another city, or make any other major life changes. Give yourself a chance to grieve for a few months, then it might be the right thing to do.

## Realize This Pain Will Subside

The death of your pet can be like a wound to your emotional self, and the pain can be very hard to face. Know that those who have gone through this experience, and who have loved their companion animals as you loved yours, report that although you will still miss your pet, the severe anguish will, eventually, subside. Things

will get better. That can help when you are in the midst
of grieving.

## Find Out Why Your Pet Died

Sometimes it can be very helpful, not only in aiding
your grieving process, but also to protect your family's
health and the health of any other companion animals,
to find out exactly why the animal died.

Of course, you or the veterinarian may know why the
pet died. But if the animal was not diagnosed and the
vet really isn't sure why it died, a ''necropsy'' can be a
good idea. This is an examination of the animal after
death that reveals the cause of death. The veterinarian
may also call the procedure an ''autopsy'' or a ''post-
mortem.''

Yes, the idea of a necropsy can be very distressing,
but it is important to protect those who are still living
and to avoid any possible health threats. Once the examination is complete, you can go ahead and honor your
companion animal with a simple or elaborate ceremony
and care for the remains in the way that you have selected. (See Chapter Eight on caring for your pet's remains.)

You may be able to request a cosmetic necropsy if
you wish the animal's body to be returned to you for
burial; however, this choice could inhibit the discovery
of the true cause of death.

## Don't Try to Speed Up the Grief Process

Your grief may last a few weeks or months or as long
as a year or more. (It should subside from the extreme

intensity of the grief you feel immediately after the death of your pet.)

But it's important to realize that you can't rush through the grief process, just because you don't like it or you don't feel it is productive. The problem with grieving is if you don't go through it now, when you have another loss later in life, that loss may be greatly intensified. So give yourself a break, and do know that grieving can't be rushed and cannot be put on a timetable.

## Change Your Routine

Very often you will have created patterns associated with your pet; for example, you always walked your dog right after work or you played with your rabbit at a certain time of day.

If the pattern was a routine one between you and your pet, then it's a good idea to substitute another activity. Rather than sit and suffer over what you cannot do, do something else. Read a book, take a walk, call a friend. Do something that *you* enjoy.

You may also wish to start changes of your routine *before* your animal companion dies if you know that he or she is terminally ill, in an attempt to prepare yourself.

After your animal's death, you may still wish to take walks as you did before with your animal, but take them at a different time than usual or choose an alternative route. Changing the time pattern and/or the location of your walks can contribute to the healing process. It's not that you're denying your grief; instead you're creating ways to resolve it.

## Visit Places You and Your Pet Went to Together

Although it may also make you sad, visiting sites that you and your pet enjoyed together can help alleviate the pain. If you visited the park on special days, then you can go to the park and remember. This is different from what you did routinely with your animal, because these special sites were not part of your everyday routines.

## Sometimes Music, Art, or Journal Keeping Can Help

Listening to your favorite music helps some people with their grieving. Other people find it helpful to keep a journal of their feelings. You may also wish to paint or draw a picture of your companion animal.

Writing a poem or article about the animal can be a great creative and emotional release for many people. The ancient Greeks were very attached to their pets and often wrote poems about them after their deaths. Reading a poem or article can help too. The "Rainbow Bridge" at the beginning of this book is a healing poem, and person after person has told me that it helped them with their grief.

## Create a Photo Album

You may be able to gather pictures of your pet into a photograph album. The act of creating it as well as the opportunity to look at it later on can help ease your grieving. Cal said it helped him to create an album of all his photographs of Buttons, his much-loved cat.

"That was the best therapy for me and it gave me something I'll have for the rest of my life. It solidifies my memories of him and puts those memories in one specific place."

## Seek a Special Site for Burial

Finding a place to bury your pet can actually also be a healing experience, whether you choose a pet cemetery or your backyard. Or maybe you wish to have your pet cremated and you will keep the cremains in a special place.

Deciding on appropriate memorials or markers can also help. (See Chapter Eight for further information on caring for your pet's remains.)

## Keep Mementos of Your Pet

Sometimes the grieving process can be helped by viewing items your pet once played with or used. So don't immediately discard every one of your animal's items. One would think that keeping them would make you feel worse—but pet caretakers say that it actually gives them comfort.

When Marlene's dog Hoover died, she created her own memorial at home, framing a sympathy card a friend had sent and gluing Hoover's tag on the corner of the card. She hung the card in the kitchen and says she looks at it often.

She also said that although she disposed of all the "doggy things," she kept the dog's harness and found herself pulling it out and smelling it for the first few days after the dog was gone. "I found it useful to leave one thing that smelled like him," she says.

## Donate Money or Services to Animal Charities

Other animal lovers find it helpful to send a check in the animal's name to the local animal shelter or an animal charity. You may wish to do volunteer work at your local humane society or animal shelter. You may also choose to care temporarily for an animal who needs special care before entering a family permanently.

Elaine donated a check to the local humane society in memory of her beloved collie Suzette and she received a letter from the director asking her if she would mind writing a tribute to her dog. She was pleased to write a short article and this act also helped her to work through her grief.

## Special Ceremonies and Rituals Help

Bereavement counselor Myrna Sogalnick says that a key issue for people who come to her group is how their companion animal will be memorialized. "We don't really know what to do to put closure on the life of a very important being that shared our life and our home, often for many years," says Sogalnick. Memorializing the animal is one good way to do this. Her support group provides people with an opportunity to discuss possible options and to make a good plan.

Some pet owners have created a "candle ceremony," described on CompuServe. Grieving pet caretakers give the names of their pets to the forum leader, and each Monday, everyone involved lights a candle at their own homes. There is a preplanned service/ritual at a specific time for all to mourn all the animals that have died or are suffering.

A program or script, posted by Marion Hale and Ed Williams, is provided in the library section of the Pets Forum. The first part is called "Ceremony," and includes reading a poem and explanation. For example, "We gather together to honor and remember our animals. Tonight we join hands, hearts, and souls across the land as one large extended family to pray for our sick and dying pets and to pay tribute to our furbabies who have gone ahead to Rainbow Bridge. Someday, we will meet them again, with hugs, tears, and kisses, as we walk together, in eternity to our new home."

Next is a sort of generic prayer (with no reference to any particular religion) and then the first candle is lit. The names of the "furchildren" who have died are read, with a brief poem. (These names have been given to the person on the computer forum who is responsible for posting such information.)

There is a deadline for providing names if you want to be in a given week's ceremony, for example Sunday at 8:00 P.M. Eastern time is the current deadline on CompuServe as of this writing.

Of course you don't have to have access to a computer forum to create your own candle ceremony or some other ritual. "Have a funeral, even if it's only a simple one," advised an interviewee. "And remember that God knows even when a sparrow falls. It's nice to know that God notices your pet dying—it's a sort of social validation."

## Find Solace in Religion

You may be among the people who find comfort and solace during your grief by turning to your religious faith. For example, Ronnie said it helped him with his grieving for Louis, his parakeet, to remember the Scripture writing about God knowing even when a sparrow falls.

Of course, some people have stated that their religion caused them problems when their pet died, because they had been instructed as children that animals could not go to heaven since they had no souls. Most animal lovers really cannot accept such a premise. (This subject is covered in the section "Do Animals Go to Heaven?" in the chapter on helping children with their grief.)

Tammy assumed that her much-loved cat would go to heaven, and after talking it over with a friend, she decided to commend the soul of her cat to her deceased sister. This thought gave her a great deal of comfort. It might work for you as well.

## Help Family Members

How can you assist other members of your household to deal with your pet's death? Begin with self-acceptance of your own emotions and extend that outward.

Want specifics? One tactic is to have a family meeting and to talk about how you miss your pet. If anyone brings up negative memories of the pet, don't chastise that person. An animal—or a person—is not sainted by dying and we all have good and bad and often humorous memories of those we love. It can be very comforting to remember the funny or silly acts of a companion animal.

You could also look at photographs of the pet together and talk about special times you had together. You may wish to create a scrapbook and/or pull out and frame a favorite photograph of your pet.

Another common, and positive and healing reaction for families is to link the pet with special times in their lives and even with the whole tapestry of their lives.

For example, "We got Brownie when Susie was two years old, and now Susie is sixteen!" They may recall when the family, including Brownie, went to the beach together. Or the time they moved to the new home, and Brownie was so confused and excited. After a while family members should be able to conjure up many memories.

Experts also say that just saying the pet's name aloud a few times can be very comforting.

## Time Can Heal—If You Accept Your Grieving

You will probably always have a special place in your heart for a loved pet that has died. But after a while, maybe weeks, maybe many months, you will be able to think of your pet with fondness and will not burst into tears or become very depressed. "It gets better eventually," said the owner of Webster, a parakeet. "You can expect to get over the loss, although you will always remember your pet."

If the grief continues just as intensely for several months, you should consider talking with a pet bereavement counselor and/or attending a pet support group.

You may also choose to see a psychologist or a psychiatrist, although remember that sometimes mental-health professionals don't understand the extent of anguish a pet lover can feel when a pet dies. Be sure to ask the mental-health professional if she or he truly understands that grief over the loss of a pet can be very painful.

Says Sogalnick, "Numerous times a client will see a therapist and the therapist will start with something general, like, 'How are you today,' and the client might say, 'I'm pretty down, my dog died over the weekend.' The therapist will spend maybe two to three minutes on that and then say something like 'So what's on your mind today?' " Clearly the therapist who reacts in this manner is not understanding the importance of the animal to the person and the significance of the loss.

## How Long Does Grief Last?

Because people vary so much in their attachments to their companion animals and also in their own individual circumstances (for example, how many previous losses they've experienced, what's going on with their life now, and so forth), it's really difficult to put a time limit on grieving. Some people may recover in a few weeks or months and others will need more time.

"Give yourself at least a year," says Laurel Lagoni, codirector of the Changes program at the Colorado State University Veterinary Teaching Hospital. Lagoni says she and her partner counsel about five hundred bereaved pet owners every year.

There's a good reason for giving yourself a minimum of this one-year timetable. After a few months you may feel like you have pretty much recovered. But over the course of a year, different events you link with your past will recur—but this time without the animal.

For example, let's say that you went camping with your dog every summer and the dog died in December.

You were very sad, and then you thought you were "over" the grief. Summertime comes. "Then you set out on that camping trip and you may feel very depressed, very shaky emotionally," says Lagoni, who explains that the grief may come flooding back because you're involved in an activity that you and your companion animal enjoyed together. The grief may come back for a few days or a week and it may be very intense. It doesn't mean there's anything wrong with you—it's the normal grief process at work. Next year at this time you may again remember what it felt like to share activities with your pet—but as time passes, the good memories become stronger.

## Other Times When You May Become Upset

For a while, perhaps a long while, different things may bring your grief back to you. For example, if you and your family celebrated your pet's birthday, as many pet caretakers do, you may feel very sad when that time comes around again. You may feel sad on your own birthday, because you have been deprived of the companionship of the animal you loved.

At those times, you may wish to say a special prayer for your pet, if this fits in with your religious beliefs. Or just remembering the joy you shared with the pet may help.

Another circumstance that can renew the grief is if you see a pet that looks just like yours. You may irrationally (and momentarily) believe that lady walking her dog has kidnapped your dog—even though you saw the pet euthanized. This is a natural, albeit irrational, reaction and you should not worry that you are losing your sanity if it happens to you.

## Pet Grief Support Groups

Because so many pet lovers feel disenfranchised or not truly allowed to grieve for their pets, sometimes a pet grief support group or bereavement group can offer you valuable help. A pet support group is generally composed of volunteers and you may attend the group once or twice or become an active and regular member for months or longer.

Sometimes people actually come to the group secretly, believing that their spouses or relatives would berate them for doing something so ''silly'' or ''crazy.'' Or they may believe that their relatives would become angry or annoyed.

People who come to these groups are fellow animal lovers and they want to help each other contend with their grief and pain. What they are not, primarily, support group leaders report, are the proverbial little old lady. ''People that come to our group have families and jobs. They all deeply love their companion animals and they need a place to be understood and where people aren't going to look at them like they're weird,'' says Sogalnick. She adds, ''I have personally met some of the nicest people through this group. We're not strange, and there's nothing unusual about this. We're not psychologically dependent. It's just regular everyday people in the group.''

Such groups are found throughout the country and the numbers are growing, but there are not yet enough of them. If there is no group in your area, you may find comfort in talking with a pet bereavement hotline counselor in another area.

To find the pet support group nearest to you, contact your veterinarian. Some groups are also listed in the Appendix of this book. It is also possible that the group nearest to you may be able to tell you about a group that is even closer than they are. Ask them. You could also contact the Delta Society for a list of support groups. (Their address and phone number are listed in the Appendix.)

## Computer Services Forums

There are also groups and forums on computer services with special sections for grieving pet lovers. For example, CompuServe has three separate forums with support group sections: the ''Animals'' forum, the ''Dogs and Cats'' forum, and the ''Pets'' forum.

In general, all provide assistance to mourning pet owners as well as a wealth of practical information on a myriad of topics. These forums also have computerized ''libraries,'' and users can call up files on bereavement and other topics. Other computer services such as America Online and Prodigy also offer helpful and practical information.

These three computer resources were praised to me by interviewees. Many people might think a computer discussion is impersonal. But actually the caring and practical help that people on such forums provide are very impressive. ''I received a tremendous outpouring of love and support from people on the [CompuServe] forum as well as on Canine-L on the Internet,'' says a woman whose dog recently died. ''It was extremely comforting and still is.''

Said another interviewee, ''I found the Dogs and Cats

forum [on CompuServe] shortly before we made the euthanasia decision. The people there supported me, and offered their love, and they didn't even know me. I feel it was a support group and I don't know if I could have gotten through this without them.''

The ''Pet Board'' on Prodigy has been especially helpful to some. Said Lois, ''They introduced me to 'Rainbow Bridge' and the candles service. They and the Bridge have helped me immensely.''

People talk openly of their feelings and their sadness on these on-line services. They wonder if they'll ever feel better. Others empathize and offer advice in a very caring manner. Remember that sometimes it's easier to talk to an empathetic stranger than to your relatives or family.

## Pet Bereavement Counselors

You may also find pet bereavement counselors through your nearest veterinary college or your veterinarian. These are people who generally provide individual counseling for a fee, which may be negotiable. Sometimes counselors also lead support groups for people who need to talk about their pet loss with others. (There is usually no cost or a very minimal fee involved with a support group.) There are an estimated one hundred pet bereavement counselors nationwide, many in major cities. Some provide telephone counseling while others feel they need to see you in person in order to truly help.

Pet bereavement counselors may be therapists in private practice or people associated with a veterinary college. Yet many people are completely unaware of their existence.

Why would you see a counselor privately as opposed to attending free support group meetings?

You may be the kind of person who doesn't like participating in groups, so a support group wouldn't work for you. Or you may feel like you want to talk about the problem in private with an understanding person. Many people also wish to privately discuss euthanasia with counselors before or after making this difficult decision, while others basically need validation, and also to be told that their feelings of grief are normal. Another reason that some people prefer individual counseling is that it makes them feel too sad hearing other people's stories, especially at a time when they are feeling so very sad themselves.

Betty Carmack, Ed.D., is a pet bereavement counselor who is also a professor at the School of Nursing at the University of San Francisco. She says that most of the people who seek bereavement counseling from her are females. "But I think that's typical of our society—that women tend to go for counseling more than men." She adds, however, "The depth of feeling among the men who come to see me is just as profound."

Carmack says some people come for a few sessions while others need more counseling. She also leads a monthly support group for people grieving the loss of a pet, and says about ten people attend each month. "I think the value of a support group is that you hear other people's stories and there's a sense of universality—that you're not alone and there are other people who understand what you're going through," she says.

"Sometimes people don't feel like they're getting enough support from family and friends and they want a place where they can tell their story about their animal and how important their particular animal was in their lives. It's important to be able to express the profound sorrow and grief people are having and to know they don't have to keep it inside.''

## What About a Mental-Health Professional?

Why not just call a local psychiatrist or psychologist if you think you need help in dealing with your grief? Although they are qualified to provide counseling, one problem with mental-health professionals is that they are part of the general public, and as such, are affected by societal beliefs. Rarely do they receive any kind of training or education on pet bereavement. As a result, unless mental-health professionals are also animal lovers, they may not truly understand the depth of attachment and the serious loss that you may be suffering.

In addition, mental-health professionals often see your pain at the loss of a pet as a ''displacement'' of some previous loss, which means they think that what you are really troubled by is some issue in the past. Because, they reason, you couldn't be *that* upset by the death of an animal.

Maybe you are upset by a past loss, but maybe it is truly the loss of the pet that *is* your real problem. A good pet bereavement counselor should be able to help you determine this. And if your problem is strongly associated with past nonpet issues, then he or she may be able to refer you to another therapist or to even see you herself.

Another problem with mental-health professionals is that they tend to wish to see you over the long term, whereas you may need to see a pet bereavement counselor only a few times before you feel like you can handle the problem. You need to make it clear to the mental-health professional that you don't want long-term therapy, if this is the case.

Don't rule out the possibility of seeing a psychologist or psychiatrist, though. Seeking any counseling takes research and planning, and finding the right therapist is work. But these professionals can be immensely helpful provided they are compatible with your needs.

## Phone Hotlines

There are also call-in phone hotlines for people who want to talk to a counselor. Many are staffed by veterinary schools. Probably the best known is at the University of California at Davis. Many people who have no access to support groups or to bereavement counselors in their area find great comfort from such hotlines. (See the Appendix for a listing of some prominent hotlines.)

## Ask Your Vet If Others Can Talk to You

If there are no support groups or pet bereavement counselors in your area, ask your veterinarian if he has the names of any other bereaved people who have worked through their pain and who might be willing to talk with you. If your veterinarian can't provide any names, ask her for other suggestions. You may also consider calling a help hotline for bereaved pet owners. You may also wish to contact the nearest veterinary school in or near your state and find out if they have a phone line to provide help.

## Cards Help

About ten years ago, Hallmark introduced a line of cards for bereaved pet owners and other companies have followed suit. Many people say they derive great comfort from receiving such condolence cards. Some save these cards as special remembrances, along with a few of the pet's important items.

If nobody buys you a card, why not purchase one for yourself? It may sound silly, but don't you deserve to be comforted? A special card may help.

## Losing Your Pet Over the Holiday Season

It can be especially painful when your pet dies around Christmas or Hanukkah. Maybe the pet was a gift to you. Or maybe you just found it very difficult to join in the celebration when you are so sad over your loss.

The holidays can become stressful in and of themselves, what with people's high expectations, the family visits, and all the extra work. In fact, the holidays are often very disappointing, and some people are greatly saddened by this.

Helen recalls the importance of her mixed-breed dog Krissy during Christmas: her dog always sat on the sofa and watched the children open their presents. When Krissy died at the age of twelve, Helen found it too difficult to celebrate Christmas in the same room, so she changed the location of the Christmas tree and gifts.

Realize that trying not to think about your grief by immersing yourself in holiday planning doesn't really work. For this reason, even if it's "your turn" to plan the dinner for twenty-eight relatives, if you feel you can't handle it, then don't.

And don't accept any "guilt trips" relatives will probably lay at your doorstep. You are entitled to your grief. When you are recovered next year, you can again become an active participant in the holiday whirls.

The next few chapters discuss the different circumstances in which pets die and the particular kinds of grieving associated with them.

# 5

# *When Your Pet Dies Suddenly*

The deep sadness you feel when a pet becomes suddenly ill and dies or is killed in an accident can be more severe than the grief you feel when your pet has a long illness. Scientists have actually documented the greater intensity of grief felt by the owner of a companion animal who dies suddenly. The self-blame may be much greater as well.

Bob was intensely guilty after his collie Max ran off and was injured in a fatal accident. Max had slipped his lead, and Bob rushed off to find him. The dog had been hit by a city bus. "I saw his body in the street and a few neighbors around him," said Bob. "I leaped from the car—forget about 'park'—it went off and bumped into a tree—and I lay down with Max. It was obvious he was dead. Someone loaned me a sheet and we wrapped him up and I took him home."

It's not because you love your pet more that you grieve more. Rather, it's that the person who knows his or her pet is ill has had some chance to work through part of the grief before the pet's death. In addition, if the pet dies quickly, the caretaker is often prone to serious guilt feelings. Why did she leave the door open—

allowing the dog to run out and be run over by a truck? Why didn't he notice that the rabbit looked sick that morning. (Perhaps the rabbit did *not* look sick in the morning—sometimes an illness can progress very rapidly and fatally.)

After shock comes the reaction of alarm, with all the accompanying physical responses—rapid heartbeat, sweating, dry mouth, and others. If your pet was not yet an adult, the guilt and pain can be magnified, as you think of the life this animal might have had—and was deprived of. And the companionship you might have had. If, on the other hand, your pet has been a family member for a long time, you can scarcely believe this has happened to you.

These powerful responses make it difficult for the grief-stricken person to maintain the normal routine of life.

Amy was particularly distraught at a freak accident that happened to her pet dove Amelia. She lost a toenail and actually bled to death while Amy frantically fought to save her. She was full of guilt, albeit unwarranted, since she had done everything she could. "The death occurred in about twenty-five minutes, with obviously little warning. I think the shock is worse this way," she says. "I beat myself up for not thinking like a paramedic! In some ways, the death seemed so avoidable. But I tell myself that if quick thinking and medical skills came so easily, people wouldn't have to be trained to do it well."

By comforting herself that she could have done no more than she did, Amy has managed to deal successfully with her grief, although of course her initial reaction was to cry and wail. "The grieving immediately thereafter was so intense, I thought that I would need to be sedated to ever sleep again,'' she says. ''I think it must be particularly hard when you are trying to save your friend's life and you can't.''

Sandy said she lost her cat Mimi in a very strange way. ''On the night that my younger daughter was born, and the one night when neither my husband nor I was home—Grandma was there—our cat got her collar caught on the heat-vent knob and strangled to death right in front of my mother-in-law.'' The grandmother froze up and was unable to do anything.

It's hard to understand why these freak accidents occur—but accidents do happen and we must accept that fact.

## Sudden Tragic Illness

Just as humans sometimes succumb suddenly to a fatal ailment, so do pets.

Greta, a woman from Germany who left her two cats at a kennel over vacation came back to see her ''rather fat'' cat Nietzsche transformed into a ''bag of bones.'' She took her home and pampered her as much as possible, but the animal rapidly became weaker and weaker. After a day she took the cat to a veterinarian, who said the cat just needed some overdue shots and some vitamins, which he administered. Two days later the cat was sicker still, and could not even climb out of her basket. Greta took her to a different vet, who diagnosed the animal as having a terminal illness. Greta chose euthanasia because the cat seemed to be in so much pain.

Emma's cat Luigi died of hepatitis a week after he was diagnosed. She says, "It was the hardest thing I've ever had to deal with. I've had pets all my life, but this one was my all-time favorite. There was a rapport that just didn't exist with my other animals, even though I loved them too." A complicating factor was that Emma had had to face several human deaths in the same year. "I noticed that each successive death seemed to dredge up the emotions of all previous deaths. My grandfather also died about twelve years earlier and I never really dealt with it until I was in the midst of grieving for my cat," she says.

Luigi was in the hospital over the Labor Day Weekend and died on Labor Day. "They wouldn't let us come in then [because it was a holiday], so there was a lot of guilt that he might have realized that we'd missed a day," says Emma. "One of my biggest worries was that my cat didn't know he was loved when he died. I kept dwelling on how terrible it must have been to be alone and in pain in an unfamiliar place."

Emma was able to resolve her grief, and says, "It was only in the process of helping someone else with similar feelings that I realized that everything my cat was in his life was confident and exuberant—he was the type of animal who could win over even the staunchest cat hater—and he did. So it was a disservice to him to wonder if he doubted my love when he died." She concludes, "The most important thing to keep reminding yourself is that it really does get better. Those first few months when it seems there's no improvement are very difficult." It's also important to allow yourself to grieve in the way you need to and take as much time as you need. You also need to know that sometimes there's a lot of improvement and then you seem to take several steps back.

Jim, a bird lover who devoted a room to his seven birds, suddenly discovered his parakeet Webster had died. He describes it this way, "When I went into the bird room, there was a feeling that something was wrong. I checked on each of the birds to see if they were all right and noted that Webster was not around. I then looked carefully and found him." Webster had died.

This man says that he and his wife both experienced strong feelings of guilt over the death. "We were unable to spend more than about two minutes with our birds in each of the two days prior to his death, and that is unusual for us," says Jim. "The hardest part for me is wondering, 'Did I do something wrong?' As a paramedic, I think I've learned to deal with death over ten years, but I suspect that a lot of those doubts came crawling to the surface when Webster died."

Paul considered his cat's Katrina death to be "sudden," although the cat had been sick for about a month. "The hardest part was the fact that with all the technology available today, she had to get a disease that couldn't be cured and was past remission. And it was also hard to accept that there was absolutely nothing I could do to stop it, nor could I have prevented it."

Jim's anguish and self-blame and Paul's difficulty in accepting his cat's death are common reactions. But the fact is, we could watch our beloved animals day and night, and eventually they would die nonetheless. They are mortal, as are we.

## More on Accidents with Pets

Sometimes animals rush off to investigate something outside that intrigues them, and a tragedy occurs—they are hit by a moving vehicle. Often you must deal with your own grief and pain and, at the same time you are chastised by others for not controlling your animal.

I can still remember the terror I felt when I was twelve and my dog Butchie was hit with a glancing blow by a bus. We rushed him to the veterinarian, who cleaned him up and said that he would need months of recuperation. We put him on the back porch in our kiddie swimming pool and my parents nursed him from there.

But others are not so fortunate as I was. Their animals are killed instantly or they die soon after. Jay described his horror when, in response to his whistle, his two-year-old German shepherd, Rex, darted out into the street in order to reach him fast. Said the man, ''He was trying to show me what a good dog he was.'' The dog was hit by a car and hurt very badly.

Jay called the vet, comforted Rex, and then rushed him off to the vet's office. The dog's breathing became ragged and strained and it was clear that he was in respiratory distress. Rex stopped breathing and Jay pulled over and gave the dog CPR. It seemed to help, but then Rex shuddered and gasped and it became quite clear that he was dying. Jay remembers screaming the dog's name, as if he could bring his companion animal back to life if he yelled loudly enough. The vet confirmed that Rex was dead and reassured Jay that there was nothing more he could have done.

Jay never had a chance to ''make up'' with his dog

and to ensure that Rex knew he was loved. Or so Jay thinks. Yet I believe Rex knew he was loved. Not too many people will give mouth-to-mouth resuscitation to an animal and show as much caring and love as did Jay.

Another thing that was very hard for Jay occurred when he returned home. It was wintertime, and as he looked out the window, he saw Rex's tracks in the snow, going away from the house. But there were no paw prints coming back. "The snow didn't go away for two weeks and I had to look at those tracks every day," Jay sadly recalls.

## Other Sudden Deaths

Katie told me that although there had been no previous signs of aggression, her cat Ditto was suddenly killed by one of her dogs, a wolfhound. "I was hysterical," she recalls. "It was so fast and it still haunts me. My first instinct was to kill the dog, and I did go get my revolver, but common sense prevented me from doing it."

It took quite a while to work through this grief, partly because of guilt and partly because of partially identifying with the animal's fear. "I felt so much guilt that I had inadvertently put him [the cat] in danger and that I couldn't get to him in time. He had to be so confused and so terrified."

Through talking about the death with others and receiving the loving support of her family, Katie was able to resolve her distress, guilt, and pain. She says, "I should note that my mother and most of my friends have grieved with me for all of my pets, as did the neighborhood kids, who would come over to play with them frequently.''

Sometimes you know that your companion animal is going to die, because your pet is suffering from a very serious or terminal illness. The next chapter covers the issues involved in this situation.

# 6

# When Your Pet Dies After a Long Illness

Although it may not seem like much of an advantage, if your pet is ill you have the chance to make a plan for his death and you also will probably have the opportunity to say good-bye.

## Anticipatory Grief

Very often when you know your pet is very sick or even terminally ill, the grieving starts before the pet's death. As the pet becomes sicker, your anxiety level and grief increase. This is one way your mind and your body are attempting to prepare you for what lies ahead.

Use this time to think about the ceremonies and rituals you want to perform and to plan what you'd like to do with the remains of the pet. Take plenty of photographs of your pet and make plans for a memorial. One family had professional photographs of their elderly dog taken with the family just before the animal was euthanized for a terminal illness. They found this helped them tremendously with the coping process.

## Caring for a Sick Animal Can Take Its Toll on You

Many interviewees made great sacrifices of time and money in nursing a very sick animal back to health. For example, Lucy is blind and her thirteen-year-old guide dog Rolf has himself gone blind, is incontinent, and has other serious problems. But Lucy will not give him up and is going to elaborate lengths to make him comfortable. When she needs to go out, she takes her much younger guide dog and takes the older dog too. Lucy needs to realize that she can't cope with her own needs and with the needs of Rolf. (See more on pet grief and disabled people in Chapter Ten.)

In another case, Tom's pet squirrel Peepers became very ill with an inner ear infection that she could just not shake. ''The last few months, I didn't want to be away for more than a few hours because I was afraid she might die. She was really consuming my life. I didn't dare to go anywhere overnight.'' The minute Tom arrived home from any outing, he rushed to check on Peepers, picking her up and cuddling her. Would he have done anything any differently? No way. Every minute with Peepers was worth it.

But providing care to a very sick animal can drain a person, both physically and emotionally. Administering injections and pills and perhaps even carrying the animal about, as well as the worrying, is a tough experience for anyone.

Maybe your pet will pull through. And maybe not. You have to rely on the advice of your veterinarian as well as your own gut-level feelings. Be sure to eat and

sleep as much as you need to and don't neglect yourself.
You won't be able to care for your animal if you should
become ill yourself.

## Guilt and Relief

Sometimes after the animal succumbs to death or is
euthanized, the caretaker can feel both relief and sorrow
at the same time—relief because the animal is now beyond pain, and because the difficult and intense caregiving is at an end. But the caregiver may feel guilty about
her relief. Yet it is a normal human emotion to feel relief
at the end of a difficult and painful experience and in
no way means you are being disloyal to your pet.

Talking it out with others can often help. It's a good
idea to attend a pet bereavement support group before
your companion animal dies or to talk to a hotline counselor or a mental-health professional competent in this
area. (Your veterinarian may be able to help and the
Delta Society may also be able to provide some suggestions. Their address is in the Appendix.)

Talk to empathetic friends and relatives too. If they've
gone through the same thing, they may be able to provide you with good emotional support.

## Planning Ahead Is a Good Idea—Even If Your Pet Isn't Sick Now

It's also a good idea to think about how you'd like to
honor your pet after death, even if your pet isn't sick or
elderly now. And if your pet *is* sick and/or elderly, it is
very important for you to do so.

Yet many pet owners avoid this subject. They don't like to think about death and other "unpleasantnesses." Also, many pet owners are at least a little superstitious—thinking that if you plan ahead for your animal's death, then that will somehow make it die. This is what psychologists call "magical thinking" and it has no basis in fact at all.

The problem is that if your pet does die suddenly, it is very difficult to come up with a good plan very fast. Many pet owners are too distraught, so they may leave the decision up to the veterinarian. A week or two later, they may wish that they had not agreed to cremation for example, and instead wish they had buried the animal in the backyard or chosen some other course of action. For these reasons, planning ahead is a good idea.

Some animal caretakers take an even further step, thinking beyond their own lives and planning for someone to care for their animals in the event of the caretaker's death or disability.

Sometimes you will choose euthanasia for your pet so that your animal need not suffer a lingering and painful death. The next chapter covers many key issues in making this decision.

# 7

# *Euthanasia Is the Choice: Dealing with this Pain*

Watching your pet become more and more ill can be very hard, but veterinarians say that if your pet can still get around and obtain some enjoyment from life, there are many reasons (in addition to the fact that you love your pet!) for allowing him to die from natural causes. On the other hand, your pet may require more care than you can provide or you may fear seeing him sink deeper into pain. It's a tough choice.

Do know that just as there are people who criticize those who choose euthanasia (from the Greek words *eu* meaning ''good,'' and *thanatos*, meaning ''death''), you will probably face critics who think that you should use euthanasia. Remember, you are making this choice for yourself and your pet and not to make other people happy or impressed.

## Your Veterinarian

It's best to talk with your veterinarian in person, if possible. The time of euthanizing a pet is the one occasion when she should be very concerned about your mental state and preparedness. Remember: Your veterinarian is an animal lover. So while you are sobbing about your pet's impending death, the vet is the one who is causing the death and this can be very emotionally draining for her. She needs to have worked out that issue in her mind. Don't be surprised if the vet is also upset or distressed.

The decision for or against euthanasia is a tough one. Could I maybe try just one more thing? You wonder. Your veterinarian can be a great help on this issue, discussing with you the probability that your pet might get better, and the degree of pain your animal feels.

In addition, you will need to come to terms with the fact that euthanasia is a compassionate, not an aggressive, act. Many people have difficulty balancing the pet's severe pain with the difficulty of releasing the pet to death. After all, you've spent the pet's entire life feeding and caring for it. It's not easy to end the pet's life, even when you know your pet is suffering.

## Guilt Feelings Are Common

Many pet caretakers experience intense guilt over choosing euthanasia, not because they feel it is the ''wrong'' decision, but because they hate having to make a life-and-death decision about their pet. This is similar to and also different from the guilt you feel after the death of a pet. In this case, you are making the death occur, albeit for positive and loving reasons. Afterward you may second-guess yourself as to what you ''should'' have done.

Experts say the one way to determine if euthanasia is the right choice is to think about the activities you enjoyed with the animal or that he or she enjoyed alone.

The next thing to do is to ask yourself if your pet can still do some or even any of these favorite activities. And finally, ask yourself if you think your pet is really happy.

It's also hard because as a person who loves his pet, you don't want him to leave you and you don't want to be the one that causes him to leave you. Said author Kathleen Cowles, "Choosing to destroy an attachment figure, regardless of how humane the procedure and intent are, rarely occurs without a strong emotional response."

The important thing to do is to try hard to consider the best interests of the animal and his quality of life, setting aside your own needs.

## Stages of Decision Making

In *Pet Loss and Human Bereavement* a book oriented to veterinarians, authors Leo K. Bustad and Linda M. Hines identify six stages/reactions to the euthanasia decision.

- Frustration and ambivalence. The pet owner doesn't want the pet to suffer but at the same time doesn't want to lose the animal. These ambivalent feelings can cause considerable tension.
- Acknowledgment of suffering. Now the owner does accept that the pet is truly suffering and decides to allow the animal to be euthanized. The decision is made, but emotions still run very high.
- Anger. In this stage, children may blame parents for the death of the animal or spouses may blame each other. Or everyone may blame the veterinarian. None

of these reactions is "fair"—but they are very common stages.

- Loss. In this stage, common grief reactions of crying, sleeplessness, malaise, and others may occur.
- Guilt. Another frequent reaction to the euthanizing of a pet is a very strong sense of guilt. Couldn't you have done just one more thing? Usually the vet provides reassurance that the caretaker did indeed choose the right course of action.
- Self-protection. A final stage that many people go through is the "self-protection" stage. This is when the owner decides he or she will never ever acquire another pet because they can't bear to go through this emotional pain. Many animal lovers change their minds later on, having missed the love of a companion animal, while others choose to remain petless. (See Chapter Thirteen on how to know if you're ready for a new pet.)

## Sometimes the Animal "Lets You Know" When It's Time

Although it is very difficult to make the decision for euthanasia, some pet caretakers report that the animal may let you know in both overt or subtle ways.

"I had signs from Molly," said Sally, owner of a sixteen-year old poodle who had contracted cancer. "They were the kinds of signs that those who have known and loved and bonded with an animal can understand—that she was ready to go. I had wanted to give her a high-quality life for as long as possible, and then to let her go peacefully, without any suffering." And so she did.

Said Tina, grieving caretaker of a boxer, "I was so worried that I wouldn't know when it was time, but Merlin let me know—he had greeted me every day when I came home for eight years, and that Monday night, he didn't even try, he was so tired."

If your pet is in pain and very ill, some people might think that choosing euthanasia would be easy. They're wrong. It is very hard to make that choice, no matter how sick your animal companion is.

You may feel particularly upset if there are expensive procedures that might save your pet, but you just can't afford them. Experts say that this decision can be a complicating factor, but if you cannot afford costly surgery or other alternatives, it is not your fault. Veterinarians point out that the expensive procedures might not "work" anyway.

## Issues to Consider

Counselors and pet experts say that you should consider different factors in making your decision about euthanasia.

First, is your pet terminally ill, either from an accident or a debilitating disease?

Is your pet in severe pain that medication cannot resolve? Does your pet seem happy or miserable?

Do you have the ability to provide for all the care your sick pet needs?

And lastly, are you keeping your pet alive primarily to fulfill your own needs rather than the needs of the pet?

## Sometimes Others Don't Understand

There are cruel people out there who will say such things to you as "I would have done *anything*, no matter what the cost." This was said to one caretaker after her dog was euthanized. It made no sense to say such a thing to a grieving person. A cold stare can be a very effective rejoinder to insensitive remarks. (And do remember that sometimes people just blurt out what they are thinking, without taking into account that their comments could be hurtful.)

## And Sometimes Others *Do* Understand

Not everyone is coldhearted and unsympathetic when an animal lover's pet dies. Said Susan about what happened after the death of her beloved dog Molly, "Friends and family helped a lot. I was amazed at how supportive our friends and neighbors were. One neighbor came to see us to see if we were okay, another sent cookies, and another brought a plant over. Other friends called and sent notes and sympathy cards. Those gestures meant a lot."

## Should You Be with Your Pet When It Is Euthanized?

Sometimes people wish to be with their animals when the euthanizing is done and sometimes they don't. Veterinarians say that if you feel that you will become distraught or hysterical, you will do your pet no good in its final moments. How do you know how you will react? It's hard to predict, particularly if this is a new situation. One possible way is to envision the scene in your mind and imagine how you might react. It's also a good idea to rely on your gut-level emotions about whether or not you could handle it.

Others feel that it's important to be with the animal at the end, so that the animal will not be frightened or feel alone. Polly found a middle ground: she placed her hands on her cat Muffin and closed her eyes as the euthanasia was performed. By doing so, she didn't have to actually watch the procedure, but her pet could feel comfort from her touch.

You may also have an underlying (and unwarranted) fear that the veterinarian will sell your animal to an experimental lab. Seeing the animal actually die will allay such very common fears.

You should discuss with your vet whether you should be present when the animal is euthanized and consider your own feelings. Don't think you have to be with the animal if your best friend says it's a "must." Maybe she can handle it and you can't. Or conversely, your friends may urge you to avoid seeing the animal at the end but you may feel it is very important. You need to do what's best for you and your pet.

Carol, who was with her cocker spaniel Brownie when he died, said that he looked at her "very deeply" just before he died, as if he were trying to tell her something, and then gave out one last long sigh.

Lisa has had several pets euthanized, and she says that in some cases she was present and in some cases she was not there. "Several years ago we lost a loving a faithful companion, Mamma Cat, to breast cancer. She held in there for two years, but gradually she succumbed to the disease and, in the end, was so thin and sickly. One day I looked at her and she looked at me and I knew her time had come.

"I took her to the vet and he came into the waiting room and took her from my arms and told me to go home. Somehow, it seemed there was something missing. I went home sad and crying and feeling as if I had let Mamma Cat down somehow.

"Last year, I lost another pet to another form of cancer. This time there were treatments to try, but ultimately to no avail. I had read some articles about being there with your pet and decided no matter how painful it was to me, I wanted to be there in those final few moments.

"I called the vet to let her know it was time. I gathered Mimi's favorite blanket, looked for some catnip in the garden, and brought her best kitty friend, Kitty Joe.

"At the vet's, Joe and I were shown to an examining room and Mimi was brought in. I placed the blanket on the table and put Mimi on it. I released Kitty Joe from his carrier and the vet left us for some final farewell and then the vet came back with the drugs to hook up to the catheter.

"She explained what would happen and everything happened just as she said. Mimi slipped quietly away from us and ended her suffering.

"Afterward, the vet cried and I cried and Kitty Joe continued to lie by Mimi's side. After a few moments the vet left us for a short while. We said good-bye again and Joe and I collected ourselves for home.

"Painful? Yes, it was. But afterward, I left feeling I had done all that was possible for Mimi. As for Kitty Joe, he understood what was happening, and after I brought him home, he was fine. Had he not been there, I'm certain he would have looked for and grieved for her for weeks.

"Is this something everyone should take part in? I think it's a personal decision."

As discussed in an earlier chapter, if you've had human relatives die of a terminal illness, you may relate this to when your pet also is suffering from such an illness. Tom said he lost his mother to cancer and remembers that he could do nothing to help her, but could only helplessly watch her die. "She wanted to die so bad," he said.

On the day of her death, Tom saw his mother make a gesture that looked to him as if she were trying to smile. He asked her if that was what she was doing, and she nodded. He believes that she was smiling because she knew the end of her suffering was near. He remembered this experience when his cat Suki became very ill. Tom knew that he could release his pet from the suffering. He said that he knew that his mother was happy when he held her, but had come to terms with her death. He thought that Suki may have felt similarly.

Still, Tom went through a period of torment, wondering whether or not his pet was happy, whether or not he should allow her to be euthanized. But he did make the decision and was able to release Suki from the pain.

## House Calls for Euthanasia

Some veterinarians will perform the euthanasia at your home, but do be prepared to pay extra for this service.

You may find it more comforting to have the procedure performed at your home because you and your companion animal are in familiar surroundings and not in a sterile atmosphere of a clinic or hospital. Ask your veterinarian if he or she offers this option if you feel that it would be right for your family.

## Should Your Children Be Present?

Probably very few veterinarians nationwide would approve or agree to having children present when a pet is euthanized. Bereavement counselor Laurel Lagoni of Colorado State University says this may be a mistake. "Our knee jerk reaction in society is to try to spare our children, but then they feel left out and they feel they didn't have a chance to say good-bye. They wonder what happened," she says.

At the veterinary hospital where she works as codirector of a bereavement counseling service, she and her partner have created a "client present ceremonial euthanasia," and children of any age may attend. The key is that the children want to be nearby and understand what is going to happen. Children can be nearby, but not directly present as the pet is euthanized.

Lagoni works in advance with the pet owners to design a ritual or ceremony that occurs at the point of euthanization. She says some people wish to burn incense or candles, and on a few occasions, priests have come in to administer last rites. She says that it can be comforting to children to participate in such rituals. (See Chapter Nine for further information on talking to your children about the death of a pet.)

## Having Other Pets Present During Euthanasia

Other animals in your household are often affected by the death of a pet, and they may cry, fail to eat, and act generally depressed. (See Chapter Eleven for further information.) As a result, some caretakers believe it's a good idea to bring in your other pets when your companion animal is euthanized, if you can. For example, Lisa brought in a cat who loved her sick cat, and some vets say that this can ease the problem of your other pets spending weeks looking for their lost friends. Ask your vet if this is possible.

And use common sense—if the euthanasia is to be performed in the vet's office, limit the number of other pets that you bring to one or two. And do be very sure to get permission from the vet beforehand. Of course, this may be far more feasible if you have the procedure done at your home.

Amy took her pets into the vet's office for the euthanization, as previously arranged. "We have a nine-year-old cocker mix, Jolie. And when we had Pepper, our dalmation, put to sleep at home, Jolie was in the room." Jolie's behavior was very different from usual. "Jolie usually would have been right in the middle, wanting the attention for herself. But on this day Jolie jumped up the arm of the couch with her back to us, not looking. When it was over, I looked at her and she was watching, with the saddest eyes I have ever seen. I think she understood."

There is also a very strong argument against having your other pets present during euthanization. Most pets are very fearful of going to the veterinarian for any reason and may be so preoccupied with that fear that they would gain little or nothing from being able to see the death and know what happened. Some caretakers try to help their other animals by bringing the deceased body home and showing it to them.

## Seeing Your Pet After Death

If your pet dies in the animal hospital or if you have had the pet euthanized, it is not unusual to ask to see her body. No matter how much you like and respect the veterinarian who is handling the disposal of the remains, many people need to see the pet to know it is really gone.

In addition, if you have any residual fears about the pet still being alive, your mind will be relieved.

## After the Euthanasia—Sometimes Relief

Many people report relief when the euthanasia is over, just as some pet owners are relieved when their pet dies of natural causes after a long and debilitating illness. So much stress has been carried up to that moment. And the person may have spent weeks or months of intensive caregiving, watching the animal get sicker and sicker. The pet is now at peace.

And yet with the relief may come guilt. How can you be *glad* your pet is dead? Are you a terrible person? Understand that feelings of relief are natural, and no, you are not a bad person if you experience this emotion.

When a pet owned by a veterinarian needs euthanasia, he or she just does it, right? Wrong. They love their pets as much as you love yours, and most choose to have another veterinarian do the job. And then they cry.

Susan, a veterinarian's helper, said she had four pets who ultimately died but only one that she euthanized. She felt she should have had the first two pets euthanized, but she just didn't have the heart or the nerve.

Then when her bluetick hound Zeus became sick, Susan decided it was necessary to hold him while he died. Later, when her cat became ill, she did the same. "They were very nice," she said of the veterinarian and staff. "They handed over a box of tissues when I needed it and were just right about keeping the conversation away from too much sympathy or too much staid professionalism."

Although she noticed that her grief was very acute the first few hours after the euthanizations, she says that the emotional pain was alleviated quite a bit by spending time with her other pets.

## Some Practical Considerations

If you do choose to euthanize your pet, you should make a late afternoon or evening appointment or an appointment at a time when the waiting room will not be crowded. Then call ahead before you leave for the vet's office, to ensure that the vet hasn't suddenly become tied up with emergencies and thus has a waiting room of people.

One man said he specifically asked the veterinarian if he could enter and leave through the back entrance. "I didn't want to have to come through the front afterward because I was afraid I'd start bawling in front of everyone," he said. His veterinarian agreed.

Ask the vet if you can either prepay or be billed. You might feel especially bad about paying the bill right after the pet is euthanized.

Discuss with the vet how the pet's remains will be handled, whether you want the vet to handle it or you want to bury your pet on your property or you choose cremation and/or a pet cemetery.

If you plan to take the pet's body with you, bring a container that the pet will fit in or ask the vet if he or she can provide or recommend something. One vet says he was startled when a family brought in an old typewriter carrying case, but the animal did fit and the case was being used as a coffin. You may also choose to purchase a pet coffin.

Get someone to go with you to the veterinarian's clinic. Even if the person does not wish to witness the euthanasia, he or she may be able to drive you home if you are too upset. This should be a person who is not as attached to your pet as you are, so he or she will be emotionally able to provide you with any needed support.

Some people may decide to euthanize a pet themselves, to avoid the cost and trauma of a visit to the veterinarian. I don't believe this is a good idea at all, unless you live on a farm, where life and death are routine matters. (Even then, I think it would be very difficult for you to end your pet's life.) In addition, and looking at the practical side, you probably would not know what type of poisonous material to use on your animal nor would you know the dose, and thus you could put your animal through unnecessary pain, fear, and suffering. Such an experience could be extremely traumatic for you and your family. I advise against it.

Many times people receive great comfort from the ritual of burying or cremating their pets. The next chapter discusses these options as well as pet cemeteries and a few other unique options.

# 8

## Caring for Your Pet After Death

Many bereaved pet owners find that a funeral or some other ritual greatly helps with the grieving process. It's a chance to acknowledge the love and importance of the pet in their lives and also to provide a sense of closure.

Whenever possible, it's a good idea to plan ahead for what you will do when your companion animal dies, whether you want your animal buried nearby or in a pet cemetery or you prefer to have your pet cremated or have the veterinarian dispose of the remains. Generally, animals are not embalmed unless you specifically request it and pay extra.

You can probably arrange for prepayment of the cremation of your pet or for burial in the pet cemetery. Whatever plan you do make, this is one less strain you'll have when the anguished time comes that your companion animal dies.

Some people prefer to bury the much-loved pet in the backyard, taking comfort that the animal is still a part of the environment. One man said he hadn't been to a funeral for years, but he found that having a funeral for his pet was very healing.

You can create your own ritual or ceremony and your

children can participate. I still remember burying my little turtle in a box in the backyard when I was about ten years old. My sister and I were both very somber as we lay the animal to rest. You may find this prospect too painful and prefer that a caring veterinarian take care of the remains for you. Others choose to have their pets' ashes strewn in a special place. Still others choose to bury their pet in a pet cemetery, although the International Association of Pet Cemeteries in Ellenburg Depot, New York, estimates that only about 1 percent of the thousands of pets that die each year are buried in a pet cemetery. There are also some unusual options for your pet, such as freeze-drying or mummification.

## Burying Your Pet in the Backyard

Assuming that your pet is not very large and there are no city ordinances against burying your pet in the backyard, this may be the right option for you. "We buried our parakeet below the window that he used to look out and the other birds still look out of," said one man.

Also know that if you don't own your own home, but are renting a home or apartment, you don't have the legal right to bury your animal in the backyard. Ask the owner or landlord—he or she may be an animal lover too, and give you permission!

Also, check with your city or town clerk to ensure that you will comply with any regulations. This is important because if the pet was euthanized, the drug remains in their bodies after death and could contaminate the area unless the pet is properly buried.

## Some Basics

If you bring your pet home, and do not bury him right away; keep him in the coldest part of your home, such as your basement or garage, until you are ready.

Place a plastic sheet on the floor, put newspaper on top of that. You can also place a blanket on top of the newspaper before you lay your pet down. Cover your pet with a sheet, towel, or blanket. One interviewee wrapped his pet squirrel in her favorite sheepskin and kissed her good-bye before he laid her to rest. Note: The animal does not become completely cold immediately after death and you may find that the body is still warm for several hours. Don't assume this means the animal isn't really dead. It is.

Bury the pet in a grave that is at least three feet deep and in a box or some other container. Also, be sure the pet grave is more than one hundred feet from any water sources such as wells, lakes, or ponds, to avoid contaminating the environment.

Use a wooden or plastic box that can be tightly closed to protect the pet from scavengers. Your veterinarian may be able to provide such a coffin or you can purchase or make one. There are also some backyard burial kits sold by companies such as Pet Rest, which provide an airtight casket, condolence card, and also counseling material for bereaved pet owners.

If your pet dies during winter and you live in a climate where the ground freezes, you may wish to ask your veterinarian to store the animal. One problem with this is that delaying the burial can make your grief more difficult to cope with.

You could also allow the body to freeze and cover the animal with a foot or more of insulation or snow. Place the body in a shaded place or on the north side of a building so that the body will remain frozen.

Place wood or some other material over the snow to protect the animal's body from scavengers.

Veterinarians advise that if you do decide to bury your pet in the backyard, and if your pet has died at the vet's office, you should be sure to dig the grave *before* you go to retrieve your pet. It is too painful to be struggling to dig a hole while your pet lies there.

## One Man's Story

Of course, you can't always do everything efficiently and in a well-planned manner when you are grief-stricken. Barry, in a poignant letter to his daughter, described the frenzy in which he dug his dog Blue's grave, overcome with anguish at the loss he experienced.

"I never dug so deeply before," he wrote, "and I was like a crazy man, working too fast, just a digging machine feeling nothing. Down around a foot and a half deep, it started to get rocky and this meant not just shoveling. Just getting the rocks out, I broke the shovel we've had for fifteen years. Then I started to claw the rocks out with little gardening tools and my bare hands. When I was satisfied it was deep enough, though it wasn't really a warm night, I was sweating profusely and it wasn't all from the effort."

In another case, Fred buried his dachshund Suzy in the backyard next to another dog gravesite. He found it very comforting to leave a kerosene lantern burning in the backyard. For about a month afterward he made sure the light was burning by the gravesite. In the morning he'd put the light out, and in the evening he'd light it again. Fred feels this action helped him a great deal. It was his way to memorialize his pet.

## Your Veterinarian Provides Help

If you don't wish to or can't bury your companion animal in your yard and prefer not to have your animal cremated or buried in a pet cemetery, you may ask the veterinarian to care for the remains.

The animal may be cremated along with other animals or it may be buried in a mass grave. In some cases, according to the International Association of Pet Cemeteries, vets will send pets to a rendering facility, where the body fat will be used.

Should you be considering asking your veterinarian to dispose of the pet's remains, it's a good idea to ask about her usual plan for disposal. Ask for the name of the service company they use. If you receive elusive answers, you may choose to contact another veterinarian.

This is important in order to avoid later regrets, if, for example, you don't like the choice the veterinarian made. For example, weeks later, you may wish that you had the animal's cremains, but the vet may have had the animal cremated in a mass cremation and thus cannot provide your particular pet's cremains to you.

## Choosing to Cremate Your Pet

Increasing numbers of people are deciding on cremation. They reason that cremation is what they plan for themselves and so consider it a good alternative for their pets. They may also see it as "environmentally friendly." Cremation will destroy any bacteria or disease left in the animal and thus not contaminate the area.

You may choose either a mass cremation, in which your animal will be cremated at the same time as other animals, or an individual cremation, in which case your animal would be cremated alone and you could have access to the cremains, either for keeping or for burial. Check with your veterinarian to make sure both these options are available.

If you ask your veterinarian, it may be possible to see what animal cremains actually look like.

Not all veterinarians are equipped to cremate animals and you should discuss this issue with your vet. Also, you should know that an individual cremation will be more expensive than a mass one. It may be possible for you to witness the cremation. If this is important to you, be sure to ask.

Some people may decide to cremate their companion animals themselves, although you should check with local authorities before doing so. You can use coal, wood, tires, or gas as the cremating agent. Paper, leaves, and grass do not generate sufficient heat.

You may choose to bury your pets' cremains on your property or in a special place. "We had Pepper cremated and we still have her ashes," said Amy of her thirteen-year-old dalmatian. She had a unique approach to the dispersion of the cremains.

"We are going to bury some here at our house, under the apple tree and among the poppies, and we'll plant her a red primrose. Another part we will take to our favorite camping spot and scatter them there. And the third part we are saving until next year or so, when we move to the home we plan to live in until we retire.''

When Jenny's dogs—Pepsie, a fourteen-year-old sheltie; Lassie, an eighteen-year-old sheltie; and Napoleon,
a fifteen-year-old beagle—died at different times, she
had each dog cremated. Jenny then had the cremains and
the dogs' collars sewn into pillows with the dog's name
embroidered on the pillow. ''These pillows with the
ashes and collars will be put in my casket and they'll be
buried with me,'' she said, referring to her own plan for
death. This was her way of making a special tribute to
her companion animals and also dealing with her grief.

One pet caretaker said that her dog was cremated but
she did not keep the cremains. ''Instead, we created a
little memorial in our backyard that not only commem-
orates Molly, but is designed to be an affirmative statement of our respect for all of the Earth's creatures.''

Another woman chose to store her cat's cremains in
a mason jar, along with her favorite toys. On the outside
of the jar, the woman placed a photograph of the cat,
along with ribbons and silk flowers.

You may or may not choose to keep your pet's remains in an urn or special container in your home and
there are many attractive vessels available through pet
cemeteries.

## Dumping the Remains: Don't Do It

Although I am confident my readers would not do
this, there are those people who will drop off the body
of their dead animal somewhere away from home. This
is unsanitary and a troubling way to dispose of an animal
that was loved. It may also be illegal.

Do not throw the body of a small animal into a garbage bag for the trashman. Can you imagine the reaction of your child if you forget and tell him or her to take out the trash—and he sees the body of the animal? You would be not only compounding the grief but could be creating a traumatic situation.

Does flushing a goldfish down the toilet count? I think it would be better to bury any animal, including a fish. Again, flushing the fish sends a very negative message to your child. (The fish doesn't/didn't matter. It was equal to excrement.) Not everyone will agree with me on this example, of course.

## Pet Cemeteries: Pros and Cons

The advantage of a pet cemetery is basically the same advantage as for a human cemetery: it provides a last resting place for your pet and one where you can visit. There are an estimated six hundred pet cemeteries in the United States today. (See the Appendix for a partial listing.) Most concentrate on dogs, cats, and other relatively small animals, although some facilities may accept horses and large animals at a higher rate.

Often the staff at the pet cemetery handles funeral services as well, and many will pick up the animal from the veterinarian's office. Some pet cemeteries operate in conjunction with other pet businesses (such as kennels and veterinary hospitals) while others are solely dedicated to the cremation or burial of pets. Fees for a pet funeral, including the plot of land, maintenance, a casket, and any other necessities start at about $223, depending on what services and products you select. Some pet owners want a very fancy casket, viewing, and other services, which can make the cost considerable.

Another advantage to a pet cemetery is that if you've buried your pet on your land, you might someday move away. If the pet is in a pet cemetery, however, you can visit it regardless of where you move. Military people have found pet cemeteries to be a good option for this reason.

One disadvantage is that many people scoff at the idea of a pet cemetery and will tell you that such places are just a rip-off. Although some pet cemeteries do undoubtedly take advantage of people, many are run by caring people. They may also have staff who can assist you with the grieving process.

Caskets for pets are relatively inexpensive; for example, according to Dennis Hoegh, president of Hoegh Industries in Gladstone, Michigan, a major manufacturer of these items, prices range from about $10 to $300, depending on what is requested.

Other costs include the funeral service and memorials (markers) identifying that your pet was buried in this site. Memorials can be made of marble, granite, bronze, or other substances. Note: You can also purchase memorials by mail, but do know that some pet cemeteries have certain specifications that must be met for markers. Check first.

There are different kinds of memorials. For example, you may choose a flat memorial, called a "flush memorial." Or you may prefer a "bevel memorial," which is somewhat higher in the back than front. (Pet cemeteries also call them "pillow markers.") Or, finally, you may choose a monument that is above the ground and is also called a "tablet" or "monolith." This type of memorial generally requires a cement foundation for support.

Given all these choices, the services of a pet cemetery can be very simple or extremely elaborate, depending on what you seek.

Hoegh recommends that you also check on what would happen to the cemetery in the event the owners die or retire. Is there a trust fund or some provision to maintain the cemetery in that event? Although the management of many cemeteries provides for this contingency, don't take it for granted.

There are not many state laws governing pet cemeteries, but California did pass a law in 1985 specifying that land can be dedicated to pet cemeteries.

A few pet cemeteries will bury owners alongside their pets or nearby. If this is important to you, be sure to ask the cemetery if they have this capability.

## What to Look for in a Pet Cemetery

When you're acutely grieving, it can be hard to evaluate a pet cemetery, so if possible, you should try to make arrangements for your pet beforehand. Whether you can make advance arrangements or not, consider some advice from Peter E. Drown, president of the International Association of Pet Cemeteries:

• Is the pet cemetery clean and well kept? Does it look like people really care about the upkeep?
• Are the people you deal with open, friendly, and helpful, or are they secretive? Will they answer all your questions?
• Has the cemetery been there at least a few years, so it has a track record? It's not a good idea to sign up with a cemetery that opened last week.

- Is the land where the pet cemetery is situated owned by the proprietors or the corporation, and not leased or rented?
- Ask the owners or managers if they have any information or can recommend any readings on pet bereavement. If they are clueless as to what you are talking about, this is a bad sign.
- What provisions have they made for the future? Drown says this is done several ways; for example, it can be stated in the deed that the land is for the pet cemetery use only. Or it can be done by contract, and the contract between the pet owner and the cemetery should stipulate how long the area is guaranteed to remain a pet cemetery.
- Is the cemetery large enough? Experts say it should be at least five acres.

It's also a good idea to have a basic understanding of some terms that pet cemetery managers may use. For example, a "mausoleum" refers to a building in which the casket is placed, which is sealed.

A "columbarium" is a structure that exists for placement of urns that contain cremains. The compartments within the columbarium are "niches."

The "holding vault" is where the animal's body is kept until burial and is a cold room or freezer.

The "preparation room" is where the animal's body is prepared for viewing, cremation, or burial.

The "selection room" is where caskets, markers, and other related items are displayed.

The "slumber room" is where the pet is placed for the family and friends to view.

"Pre-need" refers to the case where the pet owner

has made previous provisions for burial or cremation of the animal and has prepaid for these future services.

## Other Options to Honor Your Pet

Some pet cemeteries offer the option of dedicating a tree, bench, garden, and so forth to the memory of your pet and will generally provide a plaque.

## Some Unique Options

Some pet owners choose still other options. For example, PALS in Glendale, Arizona, offers freeze-drying of your animal, which results in a similar effect to taxidermy. And Summum in Salt Lake City, Utah, offers mummification.

## Preserving Your Companion Animal Through Freeze-Drying

"I have a pet cremation service and burial service," says Katherine Heuerman, co-owner of Arizona Pet Preservation and Wildlife Taxidermy in Glendale, Arizona. "I got inquiries about it, so I started researching what needed to be done."

Heuerman says her company handles about two to three animals per month, up from one a month in 1994. She anticipates being able to do about four to six per month in 1996. Customers send their pets from as far away as Pennsylvania, California, Indiana, Montana, and Florida.

Freeze-drying (or sublimation) is actually a dehydrating process that must be done under very controlled con-

ditions. The pet is positioned according to the directions
of the owner, although most people choose a reclining
position with the eyes closed. Other positions cost more.
The average time to complete a job is four to six months.
More time is needed for larger pets.

Heuerman says that the freeze-dried pets that she pro-
duces should last at least twenty years. She recommends
that they be placed in glass cases so that they will be
protected from dirt and dust.

Cost ranges from about $400 to $2,000, depending on
the size of the pet, the position selected, and other factors. For example, a 150-pound dog that is positioned
standing and alert would cost about $2,000. A sleeping
cat with its eyes closed would be $400.

The weight of the freeze-dried pet is greatly diminished from its live weight; for example, a hundred-pound
pet will weigh only about five pounds.

One man placed a "treated" pet in his foyer and plans
to have another seated right beside him.

Heuerman also does grief support volunteer work and
says that freeze-drying is an especially good option for
pet owners who have difficulty "letting go."

Note: If freeze-drying doesn't appeal to you but the
idea of taxidermy does, then you should contact local
taxidermists. Generally, they don't actively seek out bereaved pet owners, but most should be willing to assist
you.

## Mummification Is an Option

Summum, a nonprofit company in Salt Lake City,
Utah, offers pet and human mummification. (See the Appendix for their address.) According to the company,

Jews and Christians commonly practiced mummification of pets until about 400 A.D., after which it fell out of favor. According to the company's brochures, the ancient art of Egyptian mummification is used, including wrapping the pet in fine linens that have been saturated with herbs, oils, and resins. The mummification process takes a minimum of sixty to ninety days, and the cost ranges from $4,000 to about $14,000.

The mummified pet is then placed inside a bronze "mummiform" in the likeness of the animal and the animal's body is essentially preserved. A 1992 X ray of a cat that was mummified in 1985 revealed that the bone and connecting tissue of the cat remained intact and the fur and skin continued to be in very good condition.

It is also possible for you to arrange for your own mummification so that you can be together with your pet after your own death.

Whether you decide to bury your pet in the backyard, cremated, placed in a pet cemetery, or choose one of the more unique options, experts say that it's important to have some kind of plan to memorialize and treasure your pet.

Pet funerals and rituals for pets can also be very comforting for children. Many adults don't understand that children grieve for their pets, nor do they grasp how children grieve. The next chapter is devoted to helping children deal with this loss.

# 9

# *Helping Children with Their Grief*

Children can react very strongly to the loss of a pet, although not all become visibly depressed and upset. How we explain the death to our children can help ease their pain or make it worse. Many adults remember how their parents handled (or mishandled) explaining to them the death of their pets.

Don't expect to do a perfect job and don't assume that any mistakes in explaining that you may make are going to traumatize your child for life. The primary thing to remember is that you should explain in some way that the animal has died, instead of saying the animal ran away, got sick at the veterinarian's office, or some other false explanation.

Keep in mind that your body language, voice, and overall demeanor will reveal to the child that something is wrong, even if you don't say what it is.

The problem is that you must cope with your own sorrow (which may be very profound) while at the same time struggling to figure out how to explain it all to your child.

And knowing how hard it is to accept the death of your companion animal as an adult, how do you explain it to your child? You want to be compassionate and caring but at the same time you have a natural desire to protect your child. Keep in mind that your children will learn about death and serious illness as they grow up and may already have seen dead animals lying along the road.

Here's a helpful hint: Tell the child yourself about the death whenever possible and before others impart details and (possibly) mishandle the telling and frighten the child.

Remember that grief is an experience few humans can avoid. You can try to ignore it or try to skirt around it. But most of us need to go through it. And experts say that often a child's first experience with the grief associated with death follows the death of a pet. Their ability to cope with this loss may well enable them to deal with future losses—or impair them from dealing with the losses that do inevitably come.

"You need to let the child grieve," says Barry Schwartz, a psychiatrist from Pennsylvania. "I think it helps children get ready for the idea that one day they're going to find that a classmate they know got killed in an auto accident." He believes that not offering explanations to the child and not allowing a child to grieve can be a sign of dysfunctionality in a family.

Pet bereavement counselor Virginia Miller in Oklahoma City told me about a case in which a women found her parrot dead in the morning and thought about how to explain it to her five-year-old son. She made a plan and consulted with Miller before acting on it.

The woman prepared a little casket for the parrot and told the child the animal was dead. He wanted to touch it and she let him. She and the child dug a grave, said prayers, buried the parrot, and put flowers on the grave. "This was the first death the child had ever encountered in his life," says Miller.

The child was very impressed with the experience. About a day later, he was tested in school by a psychometrist for various skill levels. He told the woman all about his dead parrot and burial, and rattled them with his tale. They came out and asked her, 'Does your child have a problem with death?' And she said, 'No, his bird just died,' " says Miller.

The woman had a difficult time convincing the tester that the child was not emotionally disturbed because he talked to them about the bird's death with great interest and candor. Yet the child was behaving normally for his age and experience level. This story is a sad indictment of our culture, when a child who is introduced to the death of a pet in a loving way is seen as sick by adults.

## Two Common Mistakes of Parents

Parents make two primary mistakes in talking about the death of a companion animal with a child. One is in expecting the child to grieve in the same manner as an adult. Children should be acknowledged as individuals and as children whose reactions may be very different from yours.

The other common mistake is to expect little or no reaction and to fail to interpret the child's behavior as grief-related. For example, anger and acting out, even if the child says nothing about the animal, may have a direct relationship to their grief over the loss.

COMMON GRIEF REACTIONS OF CHILDREN*

Apparent indifference or apathy
Excessive clinginess
School difficulties
Constant daydreaming
Fear
Anxiety
Acting out
Nightmares
Crying or sobbing
Rumination (thinking over and over about the circumstances of the animal's death)
Guilt
Anger
Moving in and out of grief
Playacting the animal's death
Drop in self-esteem
Destructive behavior
Reclusiveness or self-isolation

## Adults Remembering Their Parents' Lies

Wanda, now a grown woman, told me that she still hasn't forgiven her mother for her handling of the death of a pet. She said she actually saw her puppy get run over by a truck in front of the house—and her mother made her go to summer camp that day anyway, an emotional wreck.

*Reactions vary depending on the child's age, relationship with the animal, and other factors. Your child may experience some or none of the responses described here and still be within the "normal range" of behavior. Every person is different.

Her mother promised her a new dog for her return, despite the child's hysterical crying that she did not want one. And when she returned, sure enough, there was a new puppy waiting for her. And no talk about the dead dog. Her mother followed this pattern each time a pet died, refusing to allow her child to grieve or to acknowledge that there was any grief.

"Of course I fell in love with the new pets pretty quickly once they showed up in my life," Wanda recalls. "But in looking back, I can see that this instant-replacement stuff took its toll, because I never really had the opportunity to grieve and work through that grief for any of my pets.

"I wonder what kind of message parents are giving to their kids when they rush right out and get a new pet—it really implies that living creatures are replaceable and interchangeable, which of course, they really are not."

Jerry recalls his parents' explanations of the death of a fish, bird, hamster, guinea pig, or cat. "They simply told us what happened. They explained that the animal was in no pain and was 'happy.' I recall a conversation in which my parents told me that there was lots of room in heaven for animals because people loved them so much." He added, "I also remember my mom waking me up in the middle of the night to watch a litter of kittens be born. They wanted us to see life begin too."

Many parents find it acutely difficult to explain the death of a pet to a child. For example, Bonnie spoke of what she did when her little daughter's turtle Henry disappeared and was "presumed dead." She rushed out to the pet store to try to find a turtle just like him so she could pretend that nothing had happened at all. She wanted to spare her three-year-old any pain. But none of the other turtles looked even remotely like Henry.

"I had just gotten divorced, and this was my first major single-parent trauma, so I very maturely began sobbing hopelessly in the pet store," she recalls. "The kindly old pet-store manager took me into his office and I explained the situation."

He convinced her that it was not a good idea to try to trick her child by replacing the turtle with a look-alike and told her to allow the child to grieve and to get another pet when she felt ready. She followed this good advice.

## Making Up Explanations (Or Lies): Don't Do It

Another common error is to lie that the pet ran away or that it died in the animal hospital, when the truth is that the pet died of natural causes or an accident or the pet was euthanized. No matter how hard you try, your child may find out what really happened. And then wonder what else you have lied about.

Some parents mistakenly believe that if they tell a small child that a pet is "gone," with no explanation, or if they tell a child the animal is sick and getting better—and then it never comes back—they are saving their child from grief. Nothing could be further from the truth. If you don't provide some explanation, the child's imagination will often devise something far worse.

It is hard to see your child or children become very upset over the death of a pet. But you cannot shield your children from all or even most of the sad things in life. Rather than denying them their opportunity to grieve, you can discuss with your children the good times they had with their pet and acknowledge the pain of their loss.

Another difficult part is that parents themselves may

not have come to terms with death. Says bereavement counselor Betty Carmack, ''In our society, we're not taught to talk about death and certainly not taught to explain it.'' She says the questions children ask can be particularly hard, tapping into a parent's religious and spiritual beliefs.

If you do not talk to your child about the death of a companion animal, and instead choose to hide your grief, the child will pick up on the other signals—body language, tone of voice, even reddened eyes. And their imaginations may come up with innumerable and terrible scenarios. It's better to be honest.

## Practical Information Can Help

Often children blame themselves for a pet's death, when in fact, the pet may have died of cancer, heart disease, or an injury. You can provide your children with basic information about such illnesses so that they understand that they did not cause the animal to become ill or make it die. If you don't have such information, ask your veterinarian.

## Will Your Kids Be Mad at You for Euthanizing the Pet?

It is possible that your children will be angry or resentful that you chose euthanization for your ill companion animal. And this is probably one of the main reasons (other than causing the child emotional pain) for people not telling the kids. They don't want the children to hate them.

If the children are angry with you, try to accept this

as a natural reaction and it will generally pass. (They will be more angry if they find out that you lied to them.) Try to emphasize the positive experiences you and the children enjoyed with the animal. Explain that you wanted to release the animal from physical pain and you believed this was the only way. And allow them their anger and their grief.

## Symptoms of Grief in Children

Children who are grieving the death of a pet suffer from many of the same symptoms as bereaved adults: crying, headaches, stomachaches, and other physical ailments may occur at any age. Children may also isolate themselves from their friends and classmates and refuse to go to school. Some children exhibit hypochondriacal symptoms.

In addition, a preschool-or elementary-school-aged child who has had problems with bed-wetting in the past might find that problem recurring. Daydreaming may become prominent with children at any age, as well as apathy, anxiety, and depression. The child's self-esteem may drop.

Sometimes children will act like they don't care about a pet's serious illness, and the reason for this is often that they are hoping that if they ignore it, the problem will go away. This is a form of ''magical thinking,'' and let's face it—many adults engage in it too!

Another reason for pretending not to care is that the child, particularly a male, may believe that it is unacceptable or unmasculine to grieve. This is a culturally ingrained belief. Don't expect your son to sob in front of you, but do tell him that full-grown men who loved their pets often do cry when a much-loved animal dies. Allow him the privacy to grieve alone.

## CONSIDER YOUR CHILD'S AGE

How you tell your child about a pet's death should vary according to the age of the child, and a ten-year-old child can generally understand far more than your four-year-old. Don't presume, however, that your toddler doesn't notice the pet is gone. Parents have reported their small children searching the house repeatedly for a pet that is no longer there.

### Preschool Children

Even infants and toddlers can react to an animal's death, but probably because they are reacting to your reactions. They may act out and be generally difficult. And you can't really explain what happened: they won't understand.

Preschool children may be unable to understand the finality of death and may repeatedly ask you when the pet will be "coming back." Don't worry that your four-year-old is "in denial." He really just cannot grasp the difficult concept of death.

It's also important to understand that often young children identify with the pet. This is why it's important to avoid saying that a pet died because it was sick. (See the list of do's and don'ts in this chapter.)

Another prominent fear of young children is that of abandonment, and you should be sure to give your children plenty of encouragement as well as a feeling of continuity while at the same time recognizing and speaking of the loss.

Tell your child the truth about what happened to the animal, but avoid any gruesome details. For example, if the pet was run over by a truck and its body was very mutilated, it is not a good idea to report this to your child. Simply tell the child the pet has died.

The child needs to learn that the animal has died but should not be given distressing details that could lead to nightmares. (Sometimes children will have nightmares anyway, no matter how kindly and carefully you explain the death of the pet to the child.)

Children of this age may also act out funerals or burials and, for example, bury their dolls in the sandbox. Don't assume this behavior is morbid and rush the child off to a psychologist. Children explore subjects, sometimes very difficult ones like death, through play.

## Children Ages 5 to 9

Children who are over age five are beginning to have a grasp of death but cannot fully understand its finality until after about age nine or ten. Instead, children may personify death as a sort of ''Grim Reaper.'' They continue to fantasize that death only happens to the very old and can generally be avoided.

This is a common belief among children of this age and it's not a good idea to expend great efforts to convey the finality of death to the child. Developmentally, they will probably be unable to grasp what you're trying to convey and you may only frighten or confuse them.

Children of this age may also wish to discuss the animal's death with their friends and add many elaborate details to the story. This is normal behavior for children of this age.

## Preadolescence and Adolescence

Preadolescent children begin to understand what death is and they may be very frightened of it. You need to give them plenty of comfort and TLC. The child may suffer nightmares and appetite problems and a host of other symptoms. They may fear their own death and your death and will need reassurance. You can't tell them that they will never die or that you will never die, but you can reassure them that they and you are healthy and can expect to live many years.

Adolescents are particularly vulnerable to suffering from grief. Yet they may be the least likely to show their grief because it's not "cool" or sophisticated to cry your eyes out about your rabbit dying. Don't press them hard to talk out their feelings, but do make it clear that you are sad and you are available to talk about the pet.

Be constantly aware that how you think and feel about death may have no connection with how your child regards death. Be a very active listener. Although it's a good idea to share anecdotes and how you felt when you were his age, it's also important to listen to the child's words, observe his body language, and respond to his feelings as best you can.

You may also tell the child that you are having trouble dealing with your own grief but that you'll do your best to answer questions and help understand his feelings.

## Adolescents May Grieve More

Because teenagers are not expected to be very "huggy" with their parents, and yet they still have a need for tactile comfort, the loss of a pet can be very painful for them. Some experts have said that pets also function as a transitional object to adulthood or a comfort object—somewhat similar to the blanket that the toddler must have when it goes to sleep.

As a result, experts say that adolescents may have a more difficult time than younger children in resolving their grief over a pet's death.

## Children Grieve Differently from Adults

Experts say that it's not at all unusual for a child to sob with grief for several minutes and then stop and ask if he can go out and play. This doesn't mean the grief is gone forever. It just means that's all he can deal with for now. Some adults are confused by how children evince grief, assuming they either care too much or not enough.

Grief is not something that follows a particular prescription. It is a natural human emotion, and some of us grieve more deeply than others. Also, sometimes it is not clear how deeply people are grieving, because some people, no matter their age, don't openly convey their feelings.

## Explaining Euthanasia

If your child is under the age of five or six, you may wish merely to say that the animal died rather than going into the details of euthanasia.

But if you do believe your child can grasp, at a very basic level, the concept of death, explain euthanasia as a quick and painless procedure that ends the pet's suffering. Do not say that the veterinarian killed the pet, thus transferring any guilt and blame to the vet.

Don't ask the veterinarian to lie to your children and say the pet died in the animal hospital. Says Bill McNicoll, a vet in Lima, Ohio, "I tell perfect strangers this: Go home and tell your kids like you should be telling them." He adds, "You'd be surprised—sometimes the kids are tougher than adults."

Talk to the children about possibilities you are considering for the pet's remains, whether it's burial in your backyard or a pet cemetery, or cremation.

## Some Do's and Don'ts

Try to tell the child about the death before she hears it from someone else. Your child needs you at this time.

Grief is real: don't minimize or try to rationalize away the pain for your child. It exists.

### Reassure Children It's Not Their Fault

Many adults blame themselves for the death of a pet, so it should not be surprising that children are also likely to think their animal died because of some action or inaction on their part. Or that it is even a punishment from God or fate for bad behavior.

Children need to be reassured that the cat didn't die because they didn't do their homework or take out the garbage. Or because God was punishing them for bad thoughts, especially in relation to the animal. (For example, "Oh, why do I have to take this dumb dog for a walk. I wish I didn't have to!'')

Another reason for telling children that it wasn't their fault is that they may think that if their bad thoughts made the animal die, then bad thoughts or actions could result in the deaths of their parents or themselves. This is a terrifying thought and should be addressed directly by parents, who firmly assert that there is no justification to it whatsoever.

### Share Your Own Grief

Adults often believe they should hide their grief and emotional pain from their children in an attempt to spare them. Experts say that if you are grieving, it is a good idea to tell the child you are sad too about the loss of the pet. It can also help draw you together more and assist both you and your children with the grieving process.

So if explaining the pet's death is hard for you, tell the child this. You need not present a perfect face at all times.

And if your grief is not as deeply felt as the child's? Don't minimize the child's sorrow or tell him, "It was only a gerbil," or "You're acting like a baby!" Try to be empathetic and understanding.

If your grief seems extreme, even to you, then you may wish to handle it privately. Let the children know you are upset about the death of the pet so they don't worry that something else is wrong—that you are going to die yourself or that something terrible is going to happen.

### Don't Tell Kids the Animal Is Dead Unless You're Sure

This may seem like a strange topic, but it's based on a real mistake my husband and I made when our children were only four and five years old. We were visiting my parents and we had boarded our cat Sammy. The vet called us at my parents' house and said the cat was extremely ill and probably the only thing that would save him was an expensive operation. We really could not afford it, so the vet said he was sorry, and he offered to euthanize him.

It was a horrible decision, but we didn't want Sammy to suffer, so we chose euthanasia. We waited about a half day until we felt certain that the "deed was done," and then we told the kids the truth. Or what we thought was the truth. They cried and we cried.

But then that evening the vet called to say that Sammy had had a miraculous recovery. He had coughed up a giant hairball and was feeling fine. We were very happy that our cat was alive, but we were upset that we had put our children through unnecessary grief. (Of course they were overjoyed to find out Sammy was alive and well.) So the lesson learned here is be sure before you tell your kids about a beloved animal's death.

### Answer Questions

Your pet's death may bring up painful questions. For example, if a pet could die, could you, a parent, die also? Assure your child that you are healthy and plan to be alive for a long time. But if your child asks you outright if you will die someday, simply answer that yes, you will. All living things die.

The next logical step for a child is to wonder about his own death. Is he likely to die? Again, reassure the child that he has a long life ahead of him.

One issue to avoid is morbid curiosity. Don't provide a detailed description of how an animal is euthanized or what the pet looked like after the truck ran over him, especially if the child is preadolescent or preschool. Speak in generalities instead. "He stopped breathing and died." Or, "She died instantly."

On the other hand, children often do ask what will happen to the pet's body. Explain what you intend to do, whether you're leaving the body with the veterinarian, burying it in the backyard or a pet cemetery, or something else. If you haven't decided yet, tell the child this and discuss possible options. This can give the child a feeling of empowerment in a very disempowering situation.

### Allow the Children to Talk About the Pet

Because the death of a pet is a painful experience to acknowledge, it may seem easier to brush away a child's questions and concerns. But experts say it is far better to allow the child to talk about how he or she feels. In addition, you may wish to alert the child's teacher that a beloved animal has died so she will understand any changes in behavior or performance.

If you have photographs of the children with their pets, pull them out and let your children reminisce about the good (and sometimes annoying) behavior of their pets.

**Try to Provide Some Continuity**

Experts say that whenever possible, it's a good idea to try to maintain a child's normal schedule so they can see that life does go on, even when bad things happen. This does not mean that grief is ignored and it certainly doesn't mean you send your child off to camp if she or he is in the depths of despair over the loss of a pet.

But having a friend sleep over on the weekend or going to church or playing in a baseball game are all familiar events that can indicate to the child that there is still some order to the world.

**Get Help from Others**

You may be able to work with a member of the clergy in acknowledging the death of the pet as a significant loss. Your child's teacher has probably dealt with this issue before and may have some recommendations. The teacher may also bring the subject up in class and allow a certain amount of healing and catharsis by recognizing the child's loss.

Children's books on pet loss can help too. Ask your children's librarian for assistance and also refer to the Appendix of this book for some suggestions of caring and helpful books.

**Avoid Saying These Things to Children Younger than Adolescents**

There are common statements that many parents make to their children, possibly because their own parents made them to them. Sometimes these statements can cause more emotional turmoil and upset. Avoid the following:

"Buffy was sick and died." A young child may get the idea that if you get sick, you die. Be sure to explain that the animal was *very* sick.

"Fido went on a long journey." It sounds nice, but children are very literal and you don't want them to think they are going to die if they go on a vacation with you. Also, the child could be angry and upset that she didn't have a chance to say good-bye before the pet left.

"The vet had to put her to sleep." Two mistakes here. One is that you are implicitly blaming the vet for the euthanasia. And maybe you do! But it was really your choice. The second error is referring to death as "sleep." The child may become afraid to go to sleep lest he too die. Don't tell the child that the pet is "resting" either.

In one case, a child needed a minor medical procedure and became hysterical when the doctor, in an attempt to reassure him, told him he was going to give him some medicine to "put him to sleep." It took a great deal of explaining before the child realized the doctor was not going to end his life.

A similar error is to tell the child that "Kitty is on an eternal sleep." Again, don't make sleep equal death in the child's mind.

"The cat ran away because he wasn't happy" is the wrong thing to say if what really happened was the cat died naturally or was euthanized. Don't lie to your children. This explanation can also make the child feel rejected and abandoned—after all, *why* wasn't the pet happy? Was it the child's fault? The child will wonder, even if he or she doesn't verbalize this question.

"We loved him so we let him go." This statement can be very frightening to a child. After all, you love *him*, so does that mean you could let him go? Or worse, make him die? Maybe if he misbehaves too much. These are certainly not ideas you want to convey to your child.

Instead, emphasize that the pet was very very old (if it was) and very very sick or hurt (if it was). Thus death released the pet from pain.

"God took him." Or "God took him because he was good." This makes God sound very ominous, as if He could suddenly swoop down and take a person. This is a very threatening thought for a child. And God took him *because* he was good? Does this mean you should be bad so God won't take you? This is the simple reasoning that many children would use.

Instead, if you are religious, it is far better to say that the animal died and then went to live with God.

When you say, "He was taken," the explanation is more mysterious than "God took him." The child wonders, by whom? Why? Am I in danger? What should I do?

"He passed on." To where? And why? This euphemistic explanation only begs a lot of questions from children, who are very literal-minded. Don't use it.

### Don't Fear the "D-Word"

Experts say that parents are often afraid of using the word "death" because it sounds too frightening. They want to shelter their children, which is why they use phrases like "went to sleep" and so on. But our children do see death, on television and in real life. They see animals run over in the streets and they know death happens. They may not fully understand it and it's your job as a parent to try to explain.

## Helping Your Child Express Feelings

It may help a young child to draw a picture of the animal. Older children can write down their feelings or even write a poem or tribute to the pet. (Adults find this to be very helpful too.) And be sure to tell your child, whatever his or her age, that sad feelings are normal for someone whose pet has died. Crying is normal. Feeling upset is normal. Explain that these very sad feelings will subside after a while, although the child may always remember the pet and the good times they shared.

## Do Pets Go to Heaven?

Some children—and adults—worry over what happens to the animal's soul when it dies. That is, if you believe in heaven, can you be assured that your pet will meet you there? Although this question may sound silly to some, to others it's a distressing consideration.

There is no way to know what happens after death and some theologians would argue that animals can't go to heaven because they don't have souls. Each reader will have her own beliefs regarding life after death.

The idea of a pet going to heaven can be very comforting to children and adults, and envisioning the very sick pet as now romping about in a field up there in heaven is a positive image.

Barbara remembers that when she was about ten, a friend's dog died and she was terribly upset. At chapel that morning, the Episcopal priest was talking about animals. When one of the children asked him if animals go to heaven, he answered that if they didn't, then he didn't want to go there either. Barbara says, "Perhaps this was not theologically sound, but it made us all feel better, and for some reason, it has stuck with me all this time."

Mary continued to be bothered by whether animals go to heaven from her childhood and into adulthood. "The hardest thing for me about losing my animal companions has been getting past the nuns telling me that animals don't have souls and when they are dead, they are gone." She continues, "I no longer believe this and a sense of the continuity and connection of all things helps me deal with this grief."

Maybe animals DO have a "soul." Dennis Hoegh, president of Hoegh Industries, a pet casketmaker, is collecting tales from former pet caretakers. He reports on a case of a man in Arizona who recently swore that one night when he was sleeping, his dog repeatedly licked his face. Half-awake, he ignored it at first, but the dog was very insistent about waking him up. The man did wake up and instantly smelled gas. The dog had saved his life. Only the dog had died a year earlier. . . .

Some people are also convinced that their animals play other roles after death. For example, the deceased pet somehow "sends" a new animal into the bereaved person's life, because it "knows" the person needs this companionship. Some people also believe that a pet who has died has been reincarnated into their new pet. There is no way to prove or disprove such beliefs.

## Rituals Can Help

Just as they can help adults, rituals such as funerals or ceremonies can help children obtain closure in their grief. In fact, such ceremonies may be especially meaningful for children. John recalls when his two sons, then ages fourteen and fifteen, were worried about their cat Missy. Missy was thirteen and had been in their family since the boys were toddlers. They went in search of her and found her. She had died.

Both boys were very upset, although they tried to put brave faces on and insisted on conducting a funeral. Says John, "They wrapped the body in cloth, dug a grave in the backyard, took a boom box out and played funeral music, and had a memorial service. They then buried the cat, put a rock marker on the grave, and came back inside."

In a poignant anecdote reported by a minister in a newsletter called *Caring Concepts*, Reverend Charles Hamilton describes his very first pet funeral. He happened to come across Sarah, a crying child from his church who was very distressed that her gerbil had just died.

Somewhat impulsively, he offered to conduct a funeral service at three o'clock and the child accepted his offer. He arrived at the appointed time at Sarah's house.

"There were eleven children from around the neighborhood gathered in the garage waiting for me," wrote Hamilton. "In the garage, children were standing around a foil-covered cigar box which lay in an obvious place of honor in the bed of Sarah's wagon. The wagon was draped with black crepe-paper strips and adorned with bunches of wildflowers from the vacant lot next door. Sarah had recruited her brother to be the pallbearer to pull the wagon.

"The gerbil was solemnly buried next to an oak tree and the casket was laid in the already-dug grave. Sarah laid down her flowers on top of the grave and afterward said, 'Now I know that death is really not the awful thing that I used to think it was.' "

Since then, the minister has conducted pet funerals for adults as well and says, "I have come to realize that the death of a pet . . . can be a shattering experience if not treated with love, understanding, and compassion."

## Let Your Children Talk to the Vet

Many veterinarians are very experienced in assisting families with the grief process and it may help your children to let them come in and ask the vet questions. This will clear up any mysteries in their minds.

## Is Your Child's Grieving Excessive?

Expect that a grieving child will cry, lose his appetite, and act despondent. But after several weeks and certainly months, you should start seeing improvement. If you're worried that your child is overreacting to the death of a pet, ask yourself these questions:

1. Is the anguish over losing a pet continuing to cause the child to do poorly in school, compared with past performance? After the pet's death, many children will not do as well in school because of their grief, but improvement should occur.

2. Is your child refusing to play with friends or engage in activities formerly enjoyed?
3. Do you think this grief is basically "taking over" your child? Are the usual things you do to comfort your child just not working?
4. Is your child reacting similarly to other children of the same age? Ask your friends how their children responded to the death of a pet. You may also wish to consult child-development books. If your child's reaction is far more extreme than other children of the same age, and if the child does not appear to be getting better, you may need to seek professional help.

If you do decide your child needs professional help, you don't necessarily have to rush him or her off to a child psychiatrist or psychologist. The school counselor may be able to talk out the problem with the child. Or a clergyperson may be able to help him resolve the grief and pain.

## When Is a Child Ready for a New Pet?

Psychiatrist Schwartz says parents should pay attention to the signs that a child may be ready for a new pet. For example, if you take the child to a mall and the child shows interest in looking at the animals in the pet store, this is a sign.

"If you're alert, and pay attention to what your kids say, they'll tell you when they're ready—if you listen," he says. (Chapter Thirteen addresses issues related to whether you're ready or not to acquire a new companion animal.)

# 10

## Special Needs: Disabled People and Elderly People

Dealing with your pet's death can be particularly difficult when you are a disabled person and your pet has assisted you for years. But even if your pet is not a guide dog or hearing dog, even if your pet is a "plain old" house cat, you may be housebound and as a result have become very attached to your companion animal.

If you are an elderly person whose children are fully grown and who has lost many friends, your pet may have provided you with needed love and companionship, and its death can be particularly painful.

### When a Service Animal Becomes Sick or Dies

Because animals have a shorter life span than humans, disabled people must face the loss of their animal companion and the acceptance of a new one. This poses a problem of practicality—the disabled person must adapt to a new companion, regardless of whether or not they've finished grieving over their previous one.

Also, if the animal cannot function as a service animal anymore because of illness, the disabled person may believe that somehow it is his or her "fault."

## One Man's Story

Jimmy, who has a mental disability, relies on his dog Summit when he becomes confused. But Summit has cancer, and Jimmy says his dog's illness has forced him to think about what life without him might be like. Though his coworkers and friends have raised money to pay for a needed operation for Summit, Jimmy still worries.

"I still may lose him. But it has helped so much to have the help and affirmation of friends and strangers around me, fighting to keep him alive and working. If it does pass that I should lose him, I know that there are many around me who will grieve the loss with me. I was most afraid of being alone with that grief."

## Without the Animal, Life Can Be Tough

According to a profile in *The Guideway* (published by the Guide Dog Foundation for the Blind, Inc., in Smithtown, New York), Peggy Eason found it very difficult being without a dog. The organization requires the disabled person to attend training (as do many organizations providing service animals), and for a while she was unable to attend the three week training. "It felt awful to go back to a cane," Eason reported. "I had to limit my activities and went out only when I absolutely had to, or someone went with me. I didn't feel safe without a dog. I felt very limited, which was hard because I'd become very independent."

## Other Problems

Experts say that disabled people whose animal provided assistance to them suffer the same kinds of grief as nondisabled people when the animal sickens or dies. Of course, some people are more strongly attached to their animals than others, but within the range of reactions, virtually all who lose a helping animal suffer from the shock of having to deal with their disability again on a very basic level. Now they must cope again with limitations that they had forgotten about, even something as simple as picking up something dropped, an act the dog always performed. Some people have likened the loss of the animal to becoming newly disabled.

Joan Froling of the IAADP says that another problem is that sometimes people feel their service animals are irreplaceable. She says that the person forgets that the animal had to be trained and that they must go through a learning process of adjusting to each other—that first dog did not automatically know how to get to the person's workplace or how to find the way home from the bus stop. (This is often a problem when a disabled person loses their very first assistance animal.)

In the recent past, says Froling, a disabled person's grief over the loss of an animal was ignored or ridiculed by trainers, who apparently feared that if they allowed the person to grieve openly, he or she would not bond with the new animal. Froling also says that many of the service-animal schools were created within the past decade and thus the owners, until recently, had little experience with this kind of grief.

Another problem arises when the disabled person

chooses to keep the "retired" service or guide animal as a pet and acquire a new animal to perform the jobs the "old" one did. One woman said that her older dog is very disabled with arthritis, but she is furiously jealous of the new dog, and will make a supreme effort to rush off to pick up something for her mistress.

The original dog clearly does not want the new dog to impinge on her turf, even though it's painful for her to accomplish these tasks. The owner feels very guilty seeing this, and finds it is difficult to develop a good relationship with her new dog.

## Disabled People Should Plan Ahead

Because of the importance of a service or guide animal to a disabled person, it's a good idea to plan early on for what can be done when the animal becomes too sick to work or dies.

Froling says to ask about the "successor dog policy." Some schools will not allow the person to keep a sick animal. Or if they do, they will refuse to provide another younger and healthier animal—it's one per person.

There may be a wait of not months, but years to obtain a new animal; thus you should not put off your request until your dog becomes sick (or dies). If you wait too long, you may be forced to deal with another program, and, Froling warns, some of these programs "offer poorly screened, poorly trained dogs for Tiffany prices to unsuspecting consumers."

In addition, don't just put in your application and forget about it. Check periodically to make sure it hasn't been lost.

### Elderly People Who Lose a Pet: Helping Them Cope

Animal companions can be very important to older people, improving their health and sometimes even giving them a reason for living.

In one British study, a social worker gave some of her clients birds as an incentive to keep their homes warm. Since the birds required warmth, she reasoned that the elderly people would pay more attention to the heat. She was right. That winter, none of the bird owners experienced problems with hypothermia, a common problem among her elderly clients.

Many older people dote on and love their pets, and their loss can be extremely traumatic. The elderly person may have already faced many losses—of friends and family as well as hearing or vision or mobility. In addition, the knowledge that a pet is dying or has died may cause the elderly person to consider his own mortality.

The elderly person who sees his pet as the primary (or even sole) nurturing being in his life is most at risk for severe grieving. On the other hand, it should be noted that sometimes older people are more adept at dealing with their grief, primarily because they've gone through it before. They may have lost friends, a spouse, and family members. The problem becomes most difficult when the pet caretaker is isolated and living alone and the pet may have been the only being they loved who loved them back.

The companion animal is also someone to talk to and many caretakers frequently talk to their pets. Moreover pets provide older people with a sense of order and routine. Since they are usually retired and don't have to comply with a regular schedule, many older people need the sense of orderliness, the reason to get up in the morning, that a companion animal provides.

It's also interesting to note that older people with pets are more likely to pay attention to their health, feeling responsible for someone other than themselves.

## Worry Over a Pet May Prevent Seniors from Seeking Medical Care

Experts say that often older people are afraid to go to see their physician because the doctor may require hospitalization. And who would take care of the pet? Family members and relatives should be aware of this fear and help the older person plan for it.

In addition, it's also a good idea to have the person carry a card with the name of their pets and instructions on who should be called in the event the elderly person becomes ill or some emergency occurs. The possession of this card alone could give peace of mind to an elderly person and make him or her more willing to seek out needed medical attention.

## Older People in Nursing Homes

Sometimes older people are placed in a nursing home and the staff and their relatives think they are having problems adjusting to a new place, not realizing the loss of their pet could be exacerbating the problem. Their pet may not have died, and may be under the care of a relative. Or the family may have chosen to euthanize an older pet.

Nursing-home administrators should ask new residents if they ever had a pet and allow them to express their feelings. Talking does help. Some experts recommend asking questions about companion animals on preadmission forms. If the staff knows that the new resident is upset about the loss of a pet, they can help with the grieving process.

In some cases, nursing homes are actually bringing in pets for residents to enjoy on a regular basis. Administrators have discovered the residents are happier and healthier when they have the pet's visit to look forward to.

## Getting a New Pet

The decision to acquire a new pet after grieving for a deceased pet can be especially hard for an older person, who may worry that they will be unable to care for the animal through its life. Betty Carmack, a bereavement counselor in San Francisco, says one solution is for the older person to find an older animal, usually at the local humane society or pet shelter.

"It's less likely the pet will outlive them if they bring home a seven-or eight-year-old cat," she says. And an added benefit: "Sometimes older animals are a little slower too, so they kind of fit in with their personality and lifestyle." Acquiring an older pet from a shelter can also save an animal's life.

# 11

## *Other Pets May Suffer over the Loss*

If you have other pets, they can be profoundly affected by the loss of an animal they have known for years. "Our surviving cat Alexis grieved visibly for about nine months after his death," said David. "She would pace and cry, especially at night. She didn't seem to enjoy life and became extremely dependent on us— very watchful and protective when before she was very aloof."

He continues, "Then we got another cat and she gradually went back to her old self. Now, almost two years later, she seems to be happy again.

Claudia reported that after her cat Chessie died, her other two cats stopped playing and clearly grieved for several months. In another case, a pet owner's cat became so ill that she had to be hospitalized and intravenously fed and medicated.

Donna said that after her cat Fluffy died, her two other cats would not lie down in the deceased pet's basket.

Mark said that when his beagle Toby died, his other dogs sniffed the body and watched as he held the dog before burial. "They were fairly subdued while we buried him, and didn't eat that day, but were okay after that,'' he says.

Your other pets may cry out and search for the other animal. In one case, a poodle, the daughter of the mother dog that died, howled all night after her death.

In another case, an older ferret who had essentially ''mothered'' a younger one, was very despondent after its death. She searched the house for the missing ferret until she fell down in exhaustion. For days afterward, the animal frantically searched the apartment. Afterward she checked once or twice and finally gave up.

Other behaviors may also be exhibited. The pet may ignore you or act like it doesn't like you anymore.

The pet may even behave in a hostile or aggressive manner when it had always been friendly in the past. In one case, a woman said her cat hissed at her after a much-loved ferret was euthanized. These are all symptoms of grieving.

Kathy, whose cat Huntress died after eighteen years with her, said that her other two cats were very affected when the cat became very ill. ''They spent a lot of time with her in the last few weeks she was with us. After she died, they stayed very close to me and seemed to want more attention and cuddling than usual.''

## What to Do

Your other pets will probably need some extra tender loving care for a while. On the other hand, if an animal clearly indicates it wants to be left alone, don't press yourself upon it.

You may also wish to leave the television or radio on when you go out, to provide some comfort.

If your other pets seem to become ill or refuse to eat, take them to the veterinarian. It may also help to "explain" to them what happened. They won't understand the words, but the tone of your voice may convey some comfort. But don't give your pets too much attention—you don't want to reward them inadvertently—with food or attention or both—for acting depressed or unhappy.

Try to keep your other pets to their regular routine. This helps caretakers *and* animals.

The next chapter discusses two serious losses many pet owners suffer: pets who run away and pets who are separated from their owners.

# 12

# Other Losses: Involuntary Separations and Runaways

Sometimes you have to leave your animal—or the animal leaves you. Your pet is (you hope) still alive out there, but the separation is nonetheless painful for you.

You may have to leave your animal because you're moving to a new place where they don't allow pets. Or you may develop a severe allergy to your companion animal, or marry a person who is severely allergic. Or in the worst case, your beloved animal may harm someone else and you may be forced to order him euthanized. These are a few of the situations in which you may be involuntarily separated from your pet.

## When You Must Move from Your Pet

I still remember when I was fourteen years old and my father, who was in the Air Force, was assigned to Turkey. Our family could go—but not our dog. We found a good family for him, but it was hard to say good-bye and we all often wondered how he was. I still remember that animal with great affection. Although not as painful as the grief of knowing your companion animal has died, it is painful nonetheless, knowing you will probably never see him again.

## Moving to an Apartment and Other Changed Situations

Because of changed circumstances, including a reduced income, aging, or maybe a conscious decision to cut back on expenses, you may find that you must give up your companion animal. You know that if you take an older animal to the animal shelter, it may or may not find a family (and may be euthanized). Or maybe you plan to stay in your residence, but you just cannot care for a companion animal anymore. Circumstances like becoming ill may make caring for your pet too great.

My family faced this situation with a beautiful orange cat of ours. She was extremely hyperactive, and no matter how hard we tried to train her, her personality just didn't fit with our family.

One day my husband walked from the hallway into the kitchen and happened to look up. He noticed that the cat had literally ''climbed the walls,'' and was over his head, on the wooden paneling over the door. He nearly had a heart attack.

So what did we do? We advertised in the paper for a family interested in a beautiful orange cat. And yes, we did tell the family who decided to take the cat that she was very energetic and excitable. They planned to make her an ''outside'' cat, so it worked out well for all concerned.

One interviewee told me it was very painful to retire her horse and said, ''I think that anytime you go through a change with an animal, whether it is euthanizing a pet or sending your horse to a retirement home, you want to make sure that you are in full touch with all your feelings about it.''

She continues, ''I retired my Thoroughbred last week and was as upset about that as I would be if he had died. Some people asked me how I felt as the trailer drove away. Well, I was driving the trailer. I wanted to be the one who took him to his new home. I wanted to let him go and run and have a ball. He loved it and is very happy. I am the one in mourning for my loss of this lovely guy.''

## When Your Pet Disappears

In some ways, the disappearance of a pet can be worse than its death. Although you hope to get her back, you also know that you may never see her again. Realistically speaking, you really don't know if your pet is sick or scared and you may wonder if she was stolen. Your imagination can create many frightening scenarios. And if you, an adult, can conjure up such thoughts, then think of what your child may imagine!

You feel as if you can't really grieve until you know the truth. You're stuck in an ambiguous situation, as if your pet were missing in action in a war. As a result, the ''denial'' stage of grief is extended beyond its normal duration. You may also be very angry at yourself for your own (real or imagined) negligence and you may be angry with the pet as well.

Children, especially younger ones, may become especially fearful because they often identify with their pets. They may suffer from a fear of loss or abandonment and worry about their role in the world, which is no longer seen as a safe place. They may express concern and fear that their parents can't solve this problem. So will their parents be able to protect them? Plenty of reassurance and TLC is indicated.

## What to Do When a Pet Disappears

When your pet is missing, create signs or posters and hang them up around the neighborhood and in shop windows (with the permission of the owner, of course). It's a good idea to provide as specific a description as possible: type of animal, breed, coloring, name, approximate weight, and any distinguishing characteristics. If you can provide duplicate photos, so much the better.

Go to houses in the area and ask everyone if they've seen the pet. You may also choose to advertise in the local newspaper.

Call the local animal shelters. Maybe someone brought in your pet, and you definitely do not want the animal taken by another family or, worse, euthanized.

Check "lost and found" ads in the local newspapers. It's possible you may find your pet there.

You may wish to offer a reward for the discovery and return of your pet to you, in both posters that you display and newspaper advertisements. Don't be overly lavish with the reward amount: check what others are offering for in similar situations.

You may get crank phone calls, so if anyone calls about the pet, don't let your children take the call. If it sounds like someone really has found your pet, arrange to meet him outside his house or a parking lot or possibly outside your house. Do not let strangers in your house.

Unfortunately there are thieves who will steal your pet and then seek a reward for returning the animal to you. You will probably be so grateful that you won't care. However, if you suspect that you are being victimized, contact your local police. If the scam works with you, the criminal will try it with other distraught pet owners.

In our next chapter, we'll talk about what issues to consider if you decide it's time for a new companion animal. Although much of your decision is based on pure feelings, there are also some important guidelines that you need to take into consideration.

# 13

## *When Should You Get a New Pet?*

After your pet dies, some well-meaning people may tell you to rush out and obtain a "replacement" animal. If you feel that this is a good idea, then do so. Do not, however, expect your new pet to be interchangeable with your previous one. And if you're not ready for a new pet right away—and many people are not—don't let anyone pressure you into it. So the short answer to "When should I get a new pet?" is "When you feel like it."

The problem is that if you look too hard for a "clone" of the pet you have lost, you will almost inevitably be disappointed. Even animals of the same breed have different personalities and "Rex" and "Rex Two" are bound to be very different.

Therapist Laurel Lagoni says, "When people instantly replace a loss, they're trying to circumvent the grief. What they're saying to themselves is, 'I feel lousy now and the reason is because Fluffy just died. Therefore, if I go out and get a new Fluffy, I won't feel this pain anymore.' " The problem with this reasoning is that it often backfires.

Pet lovers and experts say that it's a good idea to love an animal for itself, not for what it symbolizes to you—

137

which is the lost pet. If your new pet can't live up to your memories of the pet that died, then you may be very disappointed and your pet may not receive the love and attention it needs and deserves.

Ava was very traumatized when her bird died in a sudden accident. She wanted a new bird but felt guilty about it. So she and her husband decided they would seek out an injured bird that they could nurse back to health—rationalizing that this is what the bird that died would have wanted. They went to a pet store and discovered an ailing bird that the pet-store owner gladly gave them. In this way, they satisfied their need for a new pet with their equally pressing need to honor the memory of the one they had lost.

## It's Not Disloyal to Acquire a New Pet

Many pet owners believe that it is somehow disloyal to the memory of the pet they loved to obtain a new pet, particularly if they are experiencing guilt over the animal's death, (whether the guilt is valid or not).

If the reason why you want a new pet is to nurture and build a new relationship with it, then this is an indication that you would be a good caretaker. You would also be honoring, in a sense, your deceased pet because you are revealing the importance of pets in your life when you acquire a new animal. "I see it as a testament to a successful relationship," said one pet owner.

## How Do You Know When You're Ready?

As already discussed, it's probably not a good idea to bring home a new pet just after your pet has died (although that does work for some people). So when *is* it okay to get a new pet?

Animal lovers say you'll know. You'll find yourself drawn to the local pet store or driving by the humane society. Said Debbie, ''I waited until I could go into the humane society without bursting into tears, and until another wonderful little kitten reached out and grabbed my heart the way Marty had when I first saw him.''

You'll also find yourself noticing other people's pets and looking with interest at photos or articles of animals in the paper that need a new family—and a spark of interest is generated. Maybe that particular animal isn't for you, but you start thinking about what it would be like with a new pet.

It's probably a good idea to wait at least a month or two after the pet's death, because it may take a while for the dead pet's scent to disappear. Introducing a new pet at a time when the scent is present could prove confusing to the new arrival.

## Issues to Consider

Many people who decide they need a new pet will choose the same species, and may stick to the same breed as well. You should ask yourself several questions before you automatically search for the same kind of pet as you had before:

1. Can you love this pet for itself and not as merely a replacement of the pet who died?
2. Has your lifestyle changed? For example, if your former pet was a lively terrier, can you still keep up with a high-energy dog—or would a more se-

date dog be better for you?

3. Have your living circumstances changed? Maybe you've moved to an apartment and it would be difficult to care for a large gregarious pet. Or maybe you've moved out to the country and the big dog you've always wanted would be happy here.

4. Have your children grown up? Maybe you chose your last pet based on what you felt the children needed or could handle. If they are grown and gone, what do YOU want?

5. How much care can you provide? Do you want a high-maintenance pet or one who is more independent?

## Introduce New Pets Slowly to Old Pets

Maybe your cat and dog were inseparable and then the cat died. You should get a new cat as a friend for the dog, right? Not so fast. Animals have their own personalities and the new pet may not be a welcome addition—at least, not at first.

Experts advise that rather than bringing in a new pet permanently, caretakers introduce the animal to other pets. For example, you could try having a friend bring in the animal and ignore it yourself. Let the older pet have a chance to meet the new animal, without becoming jealous of attention you give to it.

## Some People Choose to Go Petless

Although many animal lovers will eventually obtain a new pet, there are others who feel that they can't go through all the work and pain of caring for an animal and the eventual grief of facing the pet's death. If they are fixating on the negative aspects of pet care, it is not a good idea to pressure them.

## What If Someone Gives You a New Pet—and You're Not Ready?

Many people have faced the situation in which someone who knows they've lost a beloved pet decides they really need a new one and buys one as a surprise. They may have bought into the philosophy that pets are basically interchangeable and reason it'll be fine to give you a new one. What they don't understand is the nature of pet grief.

If you are not ready for a new pet, the best thing to do is explain that you can't accept the pet. It's better for there to be some hurt feelings than for you to take on a responsibility that you don't need or want. No matter how hard you try, you may be unable to relate, and this is unfair to the new animal.

Your friend may be able to return the pet to the breeder or pet store or animal shelter. Or he may be able to find the animal another home, and maybe you could help—although it is not really your responsibility.

If you are worried that the animal will be euthanized if you turn him down, you could call the local humane society or shelter and discuss the likelihood of finding the animal a good home. Be sure to explain the situation very clearly.

## Choosing a New Pet

When people do decide it's time to select a new pet, they generally want the same kind as they had before.

In fact, it's interesting to note that many adult pet owners have the same kind of pet that they had as children.

As mentioned earlier, it's important that you don't seek an exact replica of a former pet. Even if your new pet looks just like the one that died, it is not the same and cannot be the same. Pet owners who have rushed out to buy a "clone" of their deceased pet have reported intense disappointment. Even animals of the same breed have different personalities. Don't shortchange yourself and your new pet by expecting to reenact the past.

## Factors to Consider

If you're deciding on a new pet, you should consider the following questions.

- Is your neighborhood safe for walking a pet? If you don't want to walk your animal at night, you should choose a cat, hamster, rabbit, or even a small dog who can be trained to excrete on newspapers you've laid out.
- Do you have many visitors and an active social life? If many people come to see you, with their children, you want a pet that is also friendly and outgoing and who won't have to be locked up every time that company comes.
- Are you an active person? If you are active and athletic, or at least you get out on a regular basis, an animal that enjoys the outdoors would be a good choice for you. But if you are a sedentary person who spends lots of time indoors, you will make an active pet very unhappy.
- Do you want a baby animal or a more mature pet?

Sure, baby animals are very cute. They also require a lot of training and patience. A more mature animal might be a better choice for some families.

- Do you have arthritis or some other disabling condition? If so, an extremely active pet that needs a lot of outdoors time may not be right for you. You could consider a small mammal, fish, or bird.
- Are you at home much or away from home a lot? Some animals need plenty of attention, so if you're not home very much, you should not select such a pet. In addition, some breeds of pets need a lot of grooming and care, so take that factor into consideration. For example, if you are considering a cat, you may choose to get a shorthair if you won't be around much to do the daily brushing and grooming longhaired cats require.
- Do you have any allergies to animals? Again, a longhaired cat (if you are allergic to cat dander) would be a less logical choice for you than a shorthaired cat. Or you may choose to get another type of animal altogether.
- Do you have a home business? Some people might be annoyed by animals jumping on the computer and other devices. (My cat uses my printer to jump to the top of the bookcase! She becomes quite annoyed if it is spewing out paper and she has to wait.) And of course, the animal may jump on you as well, which could be aggravating if you're trying to negotiate a big contract on the phone. (On the other hand, it might calm you down enough to cut a better deal!)
- Do you have other pets? Some animals do better as the "only child" while others can get along with your other animal companions. Don't assume a new animal

will be immediately accepted by your other pets, despite their relationship with the pet that died.

- Do you have an infant or toddler? Choose a pet that likes children and can tolerate the tail-pulling and pushing that they may receive at the hands of curious children. Be sure you don't choose a pet that would be likely to retaliate by biting. A pit bull is probably not a good match for a family with small children.

These are only a few suggestions. Be sure to ask the breeder or person who sells animals for as much information as possible on the kind of animal that you are thinking of bringing into your home. Try to find books in the library on a particular breed or type of animal before you make your decision.

## State Laws Vary on Buying/Selling Pets

You may decide to acquire your new pet from an animal shelter. Or you may instead buy from a breeder, pet shop, or private individual. As with all sales, *caveat emptor* (buyer beware). You may or may not be able to take action against the animal seller.

Be sure to provide complete disclosure if you are selling an animal yourself. Even if you do, you may get complaints, but it's still better to be up-front with information.

Some states have specific requirements for sellers of animals while others do not. It's important that you make it clear to the seller what you want and, whenever possible, put it in writing.

Also be sure to ask your veterinarian for guidance in locating an animal from a good seller. If you can, take the animal to the vet before the sale actually takes place.

State laws differ regarding the sale of pets. New Hampshire, for example, mandates that retailers who sell cats and dogs must show buyers a health certificate. California requires retailers of dogs to provide a form stating when the dog was born, its immunization record, and other health-related information. In some states, animals must have reached a certain age before they may be sold—for example, over six weeks for puppies.

Some states have laws, similar to ''lemon laws'' for vehicles, that allow the buyers to get their money back and return the animal to the seller. Such laws are in effect in Arkansas, California, Connecticut, Florida, New Hampshire, New York, Vermont, and Virginia.

Hopefully, you will have done your homework before deciding on the right companion animal for you and your family—and that this will be a long and happy alliance!

# 14

## Conclusion

One sad fact that most pet owners must face is that our companion animals will not live as long as we do, and as a result, we will have to face their deaths. It's a painful thought, and also painful for our family members. And yet by planning ahead for the inevitable and accepting death when it occurs, we can bring meaning to it all.

Many people don't understand the extreme sadness suffered by pet owners whose animals die. They may not be animal lovers or they may, in their hearts, truly understand but be afraid or embarrassed to admit it. It's okay to grieve! It's natural and it's normal.

I hope that this book has provided you with the understanding that grief is something that needs to be accepted and acknowledged, not hidden away. With such acknowledgment can also come acceptance and remembrances of past joys with your companion animal.

I hope that you have gained some key coping tactics, and that they will work for you. Sometimes one of the hardest parts of facing difficult situations is thinking that you are the only one who has ever felt this way. Know that you are not alone.

If no one in your extended family is sympathetic and understanding, there are others out there who you can talk to. It might be your neighbor, or it could be a total stranger on a telephone hotline in another state. Or a computer forum where someone from another country consoles you.

If your companion animal who has died could speak to you, I believe that he would be proud of the caring you showed through your grief and would want you to remember him and also to carry on. I hope that the information provided in this book can in some measure enable you to achieve that goal.

# Appendix

**National Organizations**

American Animal Hospital Association
P.O. Box 150899
Denver, CO 80215-0899

American Pet Products Manufacturers Association
511 Harwood Building
Scarsdale, NY 10583

The American Society for the Prevention of Cruelty to Animals
National Headquarters
424 East 92nd St.
New York, NY 10128

Animal Legal Defense Fund
1363 Lincoln Ave.
San Rafael, CA 94901
Tel.: 415-459-0885
   Note: This organization may be able to refer you to an attorney in your area with a special interest in litigation related to animals.

The Delta Society
P.O. Box 1080
Renton, WA 98057-9906
Tel.: 206-226-7357

The International Association of Assistance Dog
Partners
P.O. Box 1326
Sterling Heights, MI 48311
Tel.: 810-826-3938
   Note: Their quarterly newsletter is available for $10
   per year for assistance-dog partners and $12 for oth-
   ers. Specify whether you want print or cassette.

International Association of Pet Cemeteries
5055 Route 11
Ellenburg Depot, NY 12935
Tel.: 518-594-3000

The Latham Foundation
Latham Plaza Building
Clement and Schiller Sts.
Alameda, CA 94501
Tel.: 510-521-0920

**On-line Computer Services**

America Online
8619 Westwood Center Dr.
Vienna, VA 22182
Tel.: 703-448-8700

CompuServe
5000 Arlington Center Blvd.
P.O. Box 20212
Columbus, OH 43220
Tel.: 800-848-8199 (toll-free in United States and Canada)

Prodigy Services Co.
445 Hamilton Ave.
White Plains, NY 10650
Tel.: 914-448-2496

**Pet Loss Support Groups***

*Alaska*
Linda Bruemmer
Memories Are Forever
1206 5th Ave.
Fairbanks, AK 99701
Tel.: 907-456-7580

*Arizona*
Pet Grief Support Service Hot Line and Group
Companion Animal Association of Arizona
P.O. Box 5006
Scottsdale, AZ 85251-5006

*This is only a partial listing. There are groups that are continually forming up. Ask your veterinarian and local shelters for the names of groups in your area.

*California*
Betty Carmack, R.N., Ed.D.
Grief Counseling for Pet Owners
449 Melrose St.
San Francisco, CA 94127
Tel.: 415-334-5036

Lorri Greene, Ph.D.
San Diego County Pet Bereavement Program
2058 Oxford
Cardiff, CA 92007
Tel.: 619-275-0728

*Colorado*
Peter Poses, Ph.D., and Ruth M. Fussman, D.V.M.
The Front Range Pet Loss Support Network
1006 Robertson St. #202A
Fort Collins, CO 80524-3925

*Florida*
Maryann J. Borgon, M.Ed.
Animal Grieving Center
1408 Belle Vista Dr.
Orlando, FL 32809

*Pennsylvania*
Karen Milstein, Ph.D.
Individual and Family Bereavement Counseling
207 GSB Bldg.
Bala Cynwyd, PA 19004

*Texas*
Delta San Antonio
P.O. Box 691315
San Antonio, TX 78269

*Canada*
Pet Loss Support Group—Alberta Society
Tel.: 403-246-0091

## Hotlines

The Chicago Veterinary Medical Association Pet Loss
Support Helpline
Tel.: 708-603-3994

Pet Loss Support Hotline
University of California—Davis
Tel.: 916-752-4200

Pet Loss Support Hotline
University of Florida
Tel: 904-338-2031

Chicago Veterinary Medical Association Pet Loss
Support Helpline
Tel.: 708-603-3994

Pet Loss Support Hotline
College of Veterinary Medicine
Michigan State University
G100, East Lansing, MI 48824

Pet Group Support Service Program
Delta Society San Antonio Affiliate
P.O. Box 33265
San Antonio, TX 78265
Helpline Tel.: 512-227-4357

People Pet Partnership
College of Veterinary Medicine
Washington State University
Pullman, WA 99164-7010
Tel.: 509-335-7010
E-mail:
douglas©wsuvm1
.csc.wsu.edu

Pet Loss Support Group
WW—Madison School of Veterinary Medicine
2015 Linden Dr.
Madison, WI 53706-1102
Tel.: 608-263-7600
  Note: Many pet bereavement hotlines and support
  groups are springing up and hopefully there is or will
  be one in your area. Call your nearest veterinary college and also ask your veterinarian for assistance in
  locating a group or hotline.

**Casket and Urn Companies**

Hoegh Industries, Inc.
P.O. Box 311
Gladstone, MI 49837
Tel.: 906-428-2151

Peaceful Pets
P.O. Box 1371
Cleveland, GA 30528
Tel.: 800-422-3553

## Pet Bereavement Counselors*

*Alaska*
Linda Bruemmer
Memories Are Forever
1206 5th Ave.
Fairbanks, AK 99701
Tel.: 907-456-7580

*Arizona*
Companion Animal Association of Arizona
P.O. Box 5006
Scottsdale, AZ 85006
Pet Grief number: 602-995-5885
Organization number: 602-258-3306

Marty Tousley, R.N., M.S., C.S.
9818 E. Ironwood Dr.
Scottsdale, AZ 85258
Tel.: 602-860-6934

---

*These names and addresses were provided by the Delta Society.
Counselors generally provide individual counseling. In some cases,
name and telephone numbers only were provided. Pet bereavement
counselors may also lead support groups as well.

*California*
Betty Carmack, R.N., Ed.D.
Grief Counseling for Pet Owners
449 Melrose St.
San Francisco, CA 94127
Tel.: 415-334-5036


Lorri Greene, Ph.D.
San Diego County Pet Bereavement Program
2058 Oxford
Cardiff, CA 92007
Tel.: 619-275-0728


*Colorado*
Laurel Lagoni, M.S., and Carolyn Butler, M.S.
Co-Directors
Changes: The Support for People and Pets Program
Colorado State University
Veterinary Teaching Hospital
300 W. Drake Rd.
Fort Collins, CO 80523
Tel.: 303-491-1242


The Denver Area Pet Loss Support Group
1790 S. Bellaire St. #701
Denver, CO 80222
Tel: 303-759-1251

Peter Poses, Ph.D., MMFT, and Ruth M. Gussman,
D.V.M.
The Front Range Pet Loss Support Network
1006 Robertson St. #202A
Fort Collins, CO 80524
Tel.: 303-482-3929

*Connecticut*
Carolyn B. Allen, R.N., M.S.
504 Goose Lane
Guilford, CT 06437
Tel.: 203-453-3006

M. Patricia Gallagher, M.S.
Pet/People Needs
20 Allen-O'Neill Dr.
Darien, CT 06820
Tel.: 203-656-2669

The Omega Counseling Group
34 Argyle Ave.
West Hartford, CT 06107
Tel.: 203-588-4016

*Florida*
Maryann J. Borgon, M.Ed.
Animal Grieving Center
1408 Belle Vista Dr.
Orlando, FL. 32809
Tel.: 407-857-0190

Dora C.D. Finamore, M.S, R.P.T., C.M.P.
Tel.: 305-421-7977

*Idaho*
Patrice M. Sell
8555 Coveyridge Lane
Boise, ID 83709
Tel.: 208-362-1034

*Illinois*
Gregory Newman
The Institute for Recovery
420 Lake Cook Rd., Suite 107
Deerfield, IL 60015
Tel.: 708-680-2336, Ext. 8

Marilyn G. Putz, M.D.
Lincolnshire Animal Hospital
15820 Half Day Rd.
Lincolnshire, IL 60069

*Louisiana*
Stephanie W. Johnson, M.S.W.
Best Friend Gone Project
Office of Student Affairs/LSU School of Veterinary
Medicine
Baton Rouge, LA 70803
Tel.: 504-346-5710

*Maryland*
Carol A. Auletta
Maryland Psychotherapy Services
Tel.: 301-888-1323

*Massachusetts*
Jane N. Nathanson, C.R.C., L.R.C., L.C.S.W.
MSPCA Pet Loss Support Program
545 Ainsworth St.
Boston, MA 02131-1941
Tel.: 617-522-7400


Dorothea I. Peralta, LICSW
Tufts University School of Veterinary Medicine
Center for Animals and Public Policy
200 Westboro Rd.
North Grafton, MA 01536
Tel.: 508-839-7991


*Minnesota*
Lisette Wright
Pet Bereavement Counseling Center of Minnesota
P.O. Box 19084
Minneapolis, MN 55419
Tel.: 612-869-7702


*New York*
Paula S. Andreder
The American Society for the Prevention of Cruelty to
Animals
424 E. 92nd St.
New York, NY 10128
Tel.: 212-876-7700

Susan Cohen, M.S.W.
Director of Counseling
The Animal Medical Center
510 E. 62nd St.
New York, NY 10021
Tel.: 212-838-8100


Dr. Carol E. Fudin
Pet/People Problems
207 E. 16th St., Suite 5
New York, NY 10003
Tel.: 212-473-0932


Lucy Maynard
34 Beacon Avenue
Albany, NY 12203
Tel.: 518-458-9343


Barbara Meyers, C.G.T.
Holistic Animal Consulting Centre
29 Lyman Ave.
Staten Island, NY 10305
Tel.: 718-720-5548


Laura Schwartz, M.P.S.
64 Van Dale Rd.
Woodstock, NY 12498
Tel.: 914-679-6855

*Oklahoma*
Virginia Miller
5217 SE 82nd St.
Oklahoma City, OK 73135
Tel.: 405-672-2625

*Pennsylvania*
Ron Hathen, M.Ed, C.A.C.
Comprehensive Counseling Association: Pet Bereavement Program
717 Bethlehem Pike, Suite 1B

Linda M. Peterson, A.C.S.W., L.S.W., B.C.D.
Center for Pet Loss Counseling and Education
Sun Life Building
P.O. Box 357
Chadds Ford, PA 19317
Tel.: 610-399-3168

Barry Jay Schwartz, M.D.
Suite #214, GSB Bldg
One Belmont Ave.
Bala Cynwyd, PA 19004
Tel: 610-667-6399

*Texas*
Lynn Davidson, M.Ed., L.P.C.
Pet Bereavement Counseling Services
2400 Westheimer, Suite 209W
Houston, TX 77098
Tel.: 713-522-8344

*Utah*
Elaine A. Winter, L.C.S.W.
1414 E. 4500 South, Suite 4
Salt Lake City, UT 84117
Tel.: 801-272-9555

*Virginia*
Sandra B. Barker
Department of Psychiatry
Medical College of Virginia
P.O. Box 980710
Richmond, VA 23298-0710
Tel.: 804-828-4570

*Washington*
Susan J. Perry, MSW
7900 SE 28th St., Suite 200
Mercer Island, WA
Tel.: 206-236-4841

Gloria J. Roettger, M.S.
2633B Parkmont Lane SW, Suite H-1
Olympia, WA 98502
Tel.: 206-352-7244

**Listing of Pet Cemeteries Nationwide***

*Alaska*
Harthaven Pet Crematory
P.O. Box 2300227
Anchorage, AK 99623


*Arizona*
PALS
6051 N. 57 Dr.
Glendale, AZ 85301


Sunland Pet Rest
10917 Sunland Dr.
Sun City, AZ 85351


*California*
AA Sorrento Valley Pet Cemetery
10801 Sorrento Valley Rd.
San Diego, CA 92121


Bubbling Well Pet Memorial Park
2462 Atlas Peak Rd.
Napa, CA 94558


*This listing was provided by the International Association of Pet
Cemeteries

Franklin Pet Cemetery
2405 Ashby Rd.
Merced, CA 95340

Los Angeles Pet Memorial Park
P.O. Box 8517
Calabasas, CA 91302

My Pet's Cemetery
430 Magnolia Ave.
Petuma, CA 94952

Pet's Rest Cemetery
1905 Hillside Blvd.
Colma, CA 94014

San Diego Pet Memorial Park
8995 Crestmar Pt.
San Diego, CA 92121

Sierra Hills Pet Cemetery
6700 Vermeer Ave.
Sacramento, CA 95841

*Colorado*
Denver Pet Cemetery
57221 E. 72nd Ave.
Commerce City, CO 80022

*Connecticut*
Balmoral Pet Cemetery
P.O. Box 154
774 Kent Rd., Rte. 7
Gaylordsville, CT 06755

Forest Rest Memorial Park
2811 Hebron Ave.
Glastonbury, CT 06033


Keystone Memorial Park
Rte. 42, Cheshire Rd.
Bethany, CT 06524


Trail's End Pet Cemetery
706 Horse Hill Rd.
Westbrook, CT 06496


*Florida*
Broward Pet Cemetery
11455 NW 8th St.
Plantation, FL 33325


Cape Pet Cemetery
125 NE Pine Island Rd.
Cape Coral, FL 33909


Driftwood Pet Memorial Gardens
P.O. Box 668
800 E. Laurel Rd.
Laurel, FL 34292


Greenbrier Memory Gardens for Pets
3703 West Kelly Park Rd.
Apopka, FL 32712

Oakrest Pet Cemetery and Crematory
2845 Oakrest Place
Land O' Lakes, FL 34639


Pinellas Memorial Pet Cemetery
6505 85th Ave. N.
Pinellas Park, FL 34665


*Georgia*
Memory Gardens for Pets
1081 Dogwood Hill
Watkinsville, GA 30677


Oakrest Pet Gardens
4991 Peachtree Rd.
Chamblee, GA 30341


Savannah Pet Cemetery
P.O. Box 15847
Savannah, GA 31416


Zoophilous, Inc.
2910 Cole Court, Suite B
Norcross, GA 30071


*Hawaii*
Valley of the Temples Pet Memorial
47-200 Kahekil Highway
Kaneohe, HI 96744

*Illinois*
Fawnwoods of Windridge Memorial Park
P.O. Box 459
Cary, IL 60013


Hinsdale Animal Cemetery
6400 South Bentley Ave.
Willowbrook, IL 60514


Kozy Acres Pet Cemetery
18155 South Farrell Rd.
Joliet, IL 60432


Paw Print Garden
27 W. 150th North Ave.
West Chicago, IL 60185


*Indiana*
Peaceful Pets Cemetery
1325 Mackey Ferry Rd.
Mount Vernon, IN 47620


Union Cemetery Association
16301 North State Rd. #3N
Eaton, IN 47338


*Louisiana*
Pelican Memorials
Route 3, Box 176
Villa Platte, LA 70586

*Maryland*
Dulaney Pet Haven
200 East Padonia Rd.
Timonium, MD 21093

Friendship Pet Memorial Garden
P.O. Box 265
Waldorf, MD 20604

Resthaven Memorial Gardens, Inc.
7401 US Rte. 15N
P.O. Box 150
Frederick, MD 21701

Sugarloaf Pet Gardens
21511 Peach Tree Rd.
Barnesville, MD 20838

Valley Pet Cemetery
127 Britner Ave.
Williamsport, MD 21795

*Massachusetts*
Angel View Pet Cemetery
465 Wareham St.
Middleboro, MA 02346

*Michigan*
AAA Dog and Cat Cemetery
25280 Pennsylvania Rd.
Taylor, MI 48180

Country Meadows Pet Cemetery
11400 Demential
Demential, MI 48821


Harperlawn Pet Memorial Gardens
28600 Streamwood Lane
Southfield, MI 48034


*Minnesota*
God's Helping Hands
P.O. Box 121
Richmond, MN 56368


*Mississippi*
Pet Paradise, Inc.
4526 Office Park Dr., Suite 7
Jackson, MS 39206


*New Jersey*
Dearest Pet Memorial Cemetery
10 Letts St.
Manahawkin, NJ 08050


Petland Cemetery and Funeral Home
1155 E. Wheat Rd.
Vineland, NJ 08360


Sunset Pet Cemetery
84 Sunset Rd.
Woodbine, NJ 08270

*New York*
Hartsdale Canine Cemetery
75 N. Central Ave.
Hartsdale, NY 10530

Memory's Garden
1207 Greenwich Dr.
Albany, NY 12203

My Pet Memorial Park
10100 Church Rd.
Utica, NY 13502

Rush Inter Pet Cemetery and Crematory
139 Rush Rd.
West Rush, NY 14543

*North Carolina*
Pet Rest Cemetery
10313 Box Elder Dr.
Raleigh, NC 27613

*Ohio*
Angel Refuge Pet Cemetery
2767 Park Ave. W.
Ontario, OH 44906

Animal Kingdom Pet Cemetery
5755 Wilson Mills Rd.
Highland Heights, OH 44143

Karnik Memorial Gardens
5411 Black Rd.
Waterville, OH 43566


Woodside Pet Cemetery
6450 Shepler Church Rd. SW
Navarre, OH 44662


*Oklahoma*
Precious Pets Cemetery
P.O. Box 300
Spencer, OK 73084


*Pennsylvania*
Faithful Companions Pet Cemetery
RD #2, Box 21
Ulster, PA 18850


Golden Lake Pet Memorial Gardens
210 Andersontown Rd.
Mechanicsburg, PA 17055


Hearthside Rest Pet Cemetery
3024 W. 26th St.
Erie, PA 16506


Kimberly Memorial Park
P.O. Box 343
Fogelsville, PA 18051

Lacey Memorial Pet Cemetery
R1000 South Church St.
Hazleton, PA 18201

Pet Rest Memorial Park
RD#3, Box 464
Watsontown, PA 17777

*South Carolina*
Pet Rest Cemetery
P.O. Box 910
Goose Creek, SC 29445

*Tennessee*
Dixie Memorial Pet Cemetery
7960 Epperson Mill Rd.
Millington, TN 38053

*Texas*
Avalon Gardens Pet Cemetery and Crematory
4797 Garreth Lane
McKinney, TX 75070

Paws in Heaven
HC 3, Box 753J
Canyon Lake, TX 78132

*Vermont*
Companion Green Pet Cemetery
P.O. Box 127
Barton Rd.
West Burke, VT 05871

*Virginia*
Noah's Ark Pet Cemetery
7400 Lee Highway
Falls Church, VA 22042


*Wisconsin*
Forrest Run Pet Cemetery
N7937 Pigeon Rd.
Sherwood, WI 54169


Trail's End Pet Cemetery
N8464 County M
Algoma, WI 54201


*Canada*

Country Club Pet Memorial Park
624 147th Ave. SW
Calgary, Alberta


Sandy Ridge Pet Cemetery
P.O. Box 44
Eden, Ontario


*Australia*
The Animal Memorial Cemetery
St. Mary's Road
Berkshire Park
New South Wales, Australia

**Other Options for Care of Pets' Remains***

*Freeze-Drying*
Arizona Pet Preservation and Wildlife Taxidermy
6051 N. 57th Dr.
Glendale, AZ 85301
Tel.: 602-939-4919

*Mummification*
Summum
707 Genesee Ave.
Salt Lake City, UT 84104
Tel.: 801-355-0137

*This listing was provided by the International Association of Pet
Cemeteries

# Recommended Books and Videos For Children and Adults

## Children's Books

Samantha Mooney, *A Snowflake in My Hand*. New York: Delacorte, 1983.

E. B. White, *Charlotte's Web*. New York: Harper & Row, 1952.

Hans Wilhelm, *I'll Always Love You*. New York: Crown, 1985.

Fred Rogers, *When a Pet Dies*. New York: G. P. Putnam's Sons, 1988.

S. Sibbitt, *Oh, Where Has My Pet Gone?* Libby Press, 1426 Holdridge Circle, Wayzata, MN 55391. (This is a pet loss memory book.)

Joy Johnson, *Remember Rafferty*. Centering Corporation, 1531 N. Saddle Creek Rd., Omaha, NE 68104.

Judith Viorst, *The Tenth Good Thing About Barney*. New York: Atheneum, 1971.

**Books for Adults**

Mary and Herb Montgomery, *Goodbye My Friend: Grieving the Loss of a Pet*. Minneapolis: Montgomery Press, 1991. (This is a simple yet helpful booklet.)

Laurel Lagoni, M.S., Carolyn Butler, M.S., and Suzanne Hetts, Ph.D., *The Human-Animal Bond and Grief*. Philadelphia: W. B. Saunders Company, 1994. (Although written for veterinarians, this book is very informative and would appeal to many nonveterinarian adults.)

Herbert Nieburg and Arlene Fisher, *Pet Loss: A Thoughtful Guide for Adults and Children*. New York: Harper & Row, 1982. (Although somewhat dated, this is an interesting and helpful book for adults.)

Marvin Sussman, ed., *Pets and the Family*. New York: Haworth Press, 1985. (An intriguing look at many aspects of the human-animal bond within the family relationship.)

**Videos**

The American Animal Hospital Association in Denver, Colorado, sells a video entitled *The Loss of Your Pet*. This tape is available for $25.50 to members of AAHA and for $35.50 to nonmembers.

The Latham Foundation in California offers several videos that may be rented for a low fee ($10 if prepaid). For example, *The Human–Companion Animal Bond* is geared to junior-high students through adults. Other videos that may interest are *The Family Chooses a Pet* and *How to Raise a Puppy and Live Happily Ever After*.

Finally, the Delta Society in Renton, Washington, offers a variety of videos on pet loss for either purchase or rent.

## Bibliography

Archer, John, and Winchester, Gillian, "Bereavement Following Death of a Pet," *British Journal of Psychology* 85:2 (May 1994), 259(13).

Balk, David E., "Children and the Death of a Pet," Department of Human Development, Cooperative Extension Service, Kansas State University, April 1990.

Caras, Roger, "Saying Goodbye to Your Pet," *Family Circle* 106:13 (September 21, 1994), 164(1).

Carmack, Betty J., Ed. D., RN, "Pet Loss and the Elderly," *Holistic Nursing Practice* 5:2 (1991), 80–87.

Cowles, Kathleen W., "Loss of a Pet: Significance to the Owner, Implications for the Nurse," *Nursing Forum* 19:4 (1980), 372–377.

DeLaBarre, Michelle, R., "Pet Loss and the New Resident," *Nursing Homes* 37:4 (July-August 1988), 25(2).

Diamond, Barbara L., "Honoring a Friend," *Cat Fancy* (February 1989), 46–50.

Doka, Kenneth J., ed., *Disenfranchised Grief: Recognizing the Hidden Sorrow* (New York: Lexington Books, 1989).

Duffy, Yvonne, "Working Through Grief," *Independent Living* 8:2 (June 1993), 86(2).

Folkenberg, Judy, "Creature Comforts; Pets Cut Down Elderly's Doctor Visits," *American Health: Fitness of Body and Mind* 9:10 (December 1990), 87(1).

Friedmann, Erika, "People and Pets," *UNESCO Courier* (February 1988), 11 (3).

Froling, Joan, *Partner's Forum* 1:4.

Gaines-Carter, Patrice, "Lorton's Pet Project Tames Loneliness: Veterinarian Helps Inmates Find Caring, Responsibility with Animals," *The Washington Post* (May 2, 1988), C1.

Gerstenfeld, Sheldon L., "When a Pet Dies," *Parents' Magazine* 67:9 (September 1992), 258(1).

Hackett, Stacy N., "Healing Power: Studies Show That Pets May Help Their Owners Stay Healthy," *Pet Product News* 48:7 (July 1994), 1(3).

Harris, James, M., D.V.M., "A Study of Client Grief Responses to Death or Loss in a Companion Animal Veterinary Practice," *California Veterinarian* 36 (1982), 17–19.

Hentoff, Nat, "Lawyers for Animals," *The Washington Post* (April 28, 1990).

Hirschman, Elizabeth C., "Consumers and Their Animal Companions," *Journal of Consumer Research* 20: 4 (March 1994), 616(17).

Johnston, Joy, "Guiding Children Through Grief," *Mothering*, 51 (Spring 1989), 28(8).

Katcher, Aaron Honori, M.D., and Rosenberg, Marc A., V.M.D., "Euthanasia and the Management of the Client's Grief," *The Compendium on Continuing Education for the Practicing Veterinarian* 1 (1979), 887–891.

Kay, William J., Nieburg, Herbert A., Kutscher, Austin H., Grey, Ross M., and Fudin, Carole E., eds., *Pet Loss and Human Bereavement* (Ames, IA: Iowa

State University Press, 1984).

Keddie, Kenneth M.G., "Pathological Mourning After the Death of a Domestic Pet," *The British Journal of Psychiatry* 131 (1977), 21–25.

Kelley, Diane, Ph.D., "Coping with Grief," *Cat Fancy* (February 1989), 55–57.

Kübler-Ross, Elisabeth, *On Death and Dying* (New York: Macmillan, 1969).

Lafer, Barbara, "Helping Children Deal with Death," *Good Housekeeping* 213:1 (July 1991), 172(1).

Lagoni, Laurel, M.S., Butler, Carolyn, M.S., and Hetts, Suzanne, Ph.D., *The Human-Animal Bond and Grief* (Philadelphia: W.B. Saunders Company, 1994).

Loeffelbein, Bob, "Do Pets Affect Human Behavior?" *Pet Product News* 48:2 (February 1994), 1(3).

Lunt, Suzanne, "Easy Does It: Service Dogs for the Handicapped," *Independent Living* 9:4 (July-August 1994), 56(2).

Maggitti, Phil, "Pet Bereavement Counselors: Helping to Cope," *Cats Magazine* (August 1995), 12–15.

McClennan, Bardi, "Helping Seniors in Search for the Perfect Pet," *Pet Product News* 47:9. (September 1993), 42(6).

*Natural Health*, "Don't Take Valium, Take Your Dog," 24:1 (January-February 1994), 16(1).

Nieburg, Herbert A., and Fischer, Arlene, *Pet Loss: A Thoughtful Guide for Adults and Children* (New York: Harper & Row, 1982).

Quackenbush, James E., and Glickman, Lawrence, "Helping People Adjust to the Death of a Pet," *Health and Social Work* 9 (1984), 42–48.

Read, Susan, "A Dog's Best Friend," *People Weekly* 42:8 (August 22, 1994), 61(2).

*Research Alert*, "Pet Owners Spend As Much Time with Animals As with Their Kids" 13 (February 17, 1995), 4.

Rynearson, E. K., "Humans and Pets and Attachment," *British Journal of Psychiatry* 133 (1978), 550–555.

Segal, Julius, "Helping the Bereaved Child," *The Brown University Child and Adolescent Behavior Letter* 8:8 (August 1992), 1S (2).

Serpell, James. Ph.D., "Beneficial Effects of Pet Ownership on Some Aspects of Human Health and Behavior," *Journal of the Royal Society of Medicine* 84 (December 1991), 715–720.

Simos, Bertha G., *A Time to Grieve: Loss As a Universal Human Experience* (New York: Family Service Association of America, 1979).

Smith, Marguerite T., "The Wild New World of Health Care for Your Pet," *Money* 23:4 (April 1994), 146(10).

Stapen, Candyce H., "When Your Pet Dies," *Better Homes and Gardens* 70:10 (October 1992), 244(1).

Sussman, Marvin B., ed., *Pets and the Family* (New York: Haworth Press, 1985).

Tellem, Susan, "When You Lose a Friend," *Ladies Home Journal* 109:4 (April 1992), 126(1).

The University of California, *Berkeley Wellness Letter*, "Pet Power," 11:2 (November 1994), 2(2).

Viorst, Judith, "How Do You Talk to a Child About Death?" *Redbook* 173:1 (May 1989), 32(2).

Weisman, Avery D., "Bereavement and Companion Animals," *Omega* 22:4 (1990–1991), 241–248.

Wessel, Harry, "Strip's Farewell to Farley Reflects Reality," *The Orlando Sentinel* (April 21, 1995).

Zentay, Diana D., "Farewell to Foxy," *Saturday Evening Post* 261:1 (January-February 1989).